A Shining Season

For Ann –
May your seasons
always be shining
ones.

Love,
Mom + Dad

June 17, 1988

A Shining Season

The True Story of John Baker
As Told by William J. Buchanan

Foreword by Norman Zollinger

University of New Mexico Press
Albuquerque

To the children
and
To Polly Baker, in memoriam

Library of Congress Cataloging-in-Publication Data

Buchanan, William J., 1926–
  A shining season.

  Reprint. Originally published: New York: Coward, McCann &
Geoghegan, c1978.
  1. Baker, John, d. 1970. 2. Runners (Sports)—United States—
Biography. 3. Cancer—Patients—United States—Biography. I. Title.
GV1061.15.B35B83   1987   362.1′96994 [B]   87-19072
ISBN 0-8263-1015-X
ISBN 0-8263-1016-8 (pbk.)

Foreword

To-day, the road all runners come,
Shoulder-high we bring you home,
And set you at your threshold down,
Townsman of a stiller town.

Those lines of A. E. Housman's in "To An Athlete Dying Young" buried themselves deep in my memory more than forty years ago. They surfaced again in 1979 when I read Bill Buchanan's *A Shining Season*. Housman, had he lived in our time, could very well have been thinking of John Baker (whose shining season Bill memorializes in his book) when he penned them. Albuquerque, New Mexico was indeed a "stiller town" when John Baker died.

The story Bill tells is one of high courage. That it isn't about the kind of courage that comes in a hot, unthinking burst, as when a soldier charges a machine-gun nest, is no small part of its value. John Baker's special kind of courage required him to face, day by painful day, an enemy from whom there was no escape, and to face that enemy in a terrible war of attrition. That John could do this, while at the same time bringing a new, intensified, keener sense of life to everyone he touched in that last fateful, yes, shining season, is a story as filled with hope (in spite of the fact that there was no hope in the physical sense) as it is with anguish.

When I finished reading *A Shining Season* that November night in 1979, I mused for a while on who owed what to whom. I know Bill would be the first to admit that as an author he was in debt to John Baker, but John, too, owes something back for the way Bill told his story.

Essayist Annie Dillard makes a stunningly simple distinction between two kinds of writers. There are those, she says, who dazzle us, or try to dazzle us. "Watch my hand," they say, calling our attention to their artful manicure. The others tell us to look where they are pointing, steering us not to *them,* but to the thing which really matters—the story. Bill is that second kind of writer, self-effacing, modest, the kind of writer who respects the reader's intelligence; he makes no judgments. His prose is clear, direct, uncluttered; newcomers to *A Shining Season* will be astonished at how swiftly they are led through the John Baker story without their having missed a single important thing.

I suppose some critic, somewhere, someday, might in a careless moment call Bill Buchanan a "regional" writer.

That careless comment would be absolutely true.

He *is* a regional writer; his region is the human heart.

Bill Buchanan recognizes, as Housman did in his poem, that the death of a young runner is not an altogether tragic happening, not when what the runner leaves behind when he sets, "before the echoes fade, the fleet foot to the sill of shade," is so much more enduring, so much more a legacy for the rest of us, than the "still-defended challenge cup" he won in life.

And Bill knows, too—again as Housman did—that

> Around that early-laurelled head
> Will flock to gaze the strengthless dead,
> And find unwithered on its curls
> The garland briefer than a girl's.

Norman Zollinger

Preface

In 1975, at the urging of my two youngest children, James and Rebecca, who had been his students, I wrote a story for *Reader's Digest* about a young elementary school teacher who lived and died in Albuquerque, New Mexico. His name was John Baker. Within weeks after "John Baker's Last Race" appeared in the United States edition of the *Digest,* the Baker family and I were inundated with letters and phone calls from readers, all wanting to know more about this young man whose story had so touched their hearts. In following months, as foreign-language editions of the *Digest* were published throughout the world, these requests became international in scope. Encouraged by this gratifying reader response I put aside other projects and undertook to more deeply research the John Baker story. The result was my first book, *A Shining Season,* originally published by Coward, McCann & Geoghegan in November 1978. A paperback edition by Bantam Books was published in August 1979. In all, the book went through seven printings—a quarter of a million copies.

By far, the most (and most heart touching) letters I receive about *A Shining Season* are from young people. It is primarily for this reason that I am so grateful to the University of New Mexico Press for bringing the book back into publication. With this new edition, John Baker's story can continue to work its uplifting magic among those to whom he dedicated his life—the young.

Acknowledgments

In addition to those already named in the text the author wishes to express his deep appreciation to: Laverne and Lois Adams; LeRoy Bearman; William A. H. Birnie; Ruby Brooks; Milli, James and Rebecca Buchanan; Lisa Chiavario; Tom Clark; Robert Daugherty; Tow Diehm; Senator Pete Domenici; Clifford Donnell; Clint, Carol, Mary, Therese, Jeff and Tony Dorwart; Nancy, Beth and Chip Everett; Ken Freberg; Carolyn Freeman; John (Sr.) and Chris Haaland; Patricia Hamblett; Lowell Hickey; J. D. Kailer; Alice King; Don Kirby; Dr. Lawrence Lamb; Bob Lee; Gregory Lucero; Beverly Miller; Dr. Ward Allen Minge; Dr. Bernhard Mittemeyer; Christina Montano; Harvey, Ruth and Buddy Mynatt; Frances Hawk Nelson; Dr. T. M. Pearce; Adolph Plummer; Albert Ravanelli; Clarence Robinson; Gail Saavedra; Sharon Schul; John Sinclair; Dr. Doyle Simmons; Dr. Ernest Stapleton; Dr. Frank Papcsy; Kurt McCracken; Jim Walker; Sally, Butch, Rick, and Teddi White; Nadine Whitten; Paul Straquadine; Debbie Williamson; and others who wish to remain unnamed but whose help was invaluable during the research and writing of this book.

Author's Note

This story is true. It is recounted as closely as possible to eyewitness accounts or to John Baker's revelation of events to his family and closest friends.

A shorter version of the story appeared in *The Reader's Digest*, August 1975, under the title "John Baker's Last Race."

Chapter 1

The future looked bright to John Willard Baker that Monday, May 26, 1969. Twenty-four and at the pinnacle of a remarkable athletic career, ranked eighth among the world's indoor milers, he had fixed his dreams on the goal of competing for the United States in the 1972 Olympic Games in Munich. Before entering the Olympic trials, he vowed he would break the four-minute mile. His best time so far was 4:01.

These thoughts were on John Baker's mind at two o'clock that clear spring day as he dismissed his last afternoon class at Albuquerque's Aspen Elementary School. Minutes later, at the wheel of his compact Triumph GT–6 sportscar, he pulled away from the Aspen parking lot and headed east out of town. As he drove he concentrated on the elusive "one second." *This could be the day*, he mused. He was eager to reach his destination.

13

On the eastern outskirts of Albuquerque, just north of where Interstate 40 intersects with old Route 66, there was a high conical hill emblazoned with a gigantic whitewashed letter "U." The letter had been there for two decades in proud tribute to John's alma mater, the University of New Mexico. Fanning out in all directions from Big U Hill, the vast unfenced mesa was a boulder-strewn, windswept range of sage and cactus. It was a place where jackrabbits fed undisturbed in the afternoon shadows, where coyotes scampered wildly when flushed from their lairs. It was a place John loved. For eight years, since he had first become a competitive runner, he had come to this lonely mesa to train in solitude. Here he tested himself against the one unyielding opponent of all track champions—time.

A half hour's drive from Aspen, he parked at the base of Big U Hill and got out of his car. After fifteen minutes of warm-up calisthenics, he removed his zippered windbreaker and trousers and put them on the car seat. Beneath his outer clothing he wore his old UNM track suit. The silver-colored trunks and jersey enhanced his perpetual, deep-bronze tan. Leaning against the hood he kicked off his loafers and tightly laced on his spiked track shoes. Then, from the glove compartment, he retrieved his stopwatch. For a moment he studied it thoughtfully. He knew self-timing was crude at best. Nevertheless, it helped measure his progress.

A short walk downhill from the car he came to the starting point of his measured mile, clearly marked by the low cairns he had set in place years before. Stretching to his full height, he took several deep breaths and released them slowly. Then, planting his feet firmly beside the first cairn he knelt into his starting crouch. Slowly, he counted down: "*Five . . . four . . . three . . . two . . . one . . .*"

14

At *"Go!"* he simultaneously clicked the stopwatch to a start and kicked off in a measured pace.

It was going well. Years of hard training had honed his mind and body into a coordinated machine. Head high, exactly on stride, he calculated the time and distance remaining until the moment when he would call on all his reserve energy for the final furious sprint. That moment was near. His muscles tensed. *Now!* Suddenly, as if a giant hand had clasped him across the eyes, day turned to night. Fighting to stay on his feet he struggled against impenetrable blackness. Then his knees buckled and he sprawled forward in the dirt. An excruciating pain shot upward from his pelvis to his neck. He pushed up on his hands. and tried to rise, but he couldn't. Face down in the dirt, gasping for air, he felt his throat and lungs clog with inhaled dust. He began to cough. Panic-stricken he was seized by a terrifying thought. *My God . . . I've been shot!* Summoning all his strength he rolled onto his back and examined his body frantically with both hands. No blood, no wound. Half-blind, pain-wracked, he pulled himself into a sitting position and crawled across the rough ground to a boulder. He leaned against it and sought to control his labored breathing. In an effort to ease the sharp spasms contracting his torso, he pressed his hands firmly against his chest and screamed. The pressure intensified the pain. Sweating profusely he raised his shirt. The movement of the material across his chest was like a red-hot file on his skin. Scared, bewildered, he dropped his hands to his side and lay back against the boulder. "What happened?" he muttered aloud. Then, in anger and desperation, he shouted: "WHAT THE HELL HAPPEN-N-N-E-D-?"

He remained there, unmoving, for almost an hour. At last the pain subsided. His vision and breathing slowly returned

15

to normal. He pushed himself to his feet and found his legs were rubbery, but he could walk. He went over to where he had fallen and bent down to pick up his stopwatch. All at once the pain hit again. For a moment he wondered if he would be able to straighten up. Then, as quickly as it came, it once again subsided. With slow, even steps he walked back to his car. Not bothering to change, he climbed into the Triumph and drove away from the mesa in his track clothes.

Forty minutes later he pulled into the tree-lined driveway in front of the modest annatto brick home on Kentucky Street in the Northeast Heights section of Albuquerque where he lived with his parents. Hastily he showered and changed his clothes. But he couldn't disguise the abrasions on his hands or the ugly bruise on his right cheek.

Jack and Polly Baker both worked. Following a long and varied career, Jack, in semi-retirement, was manager of the Albuquerque Civic Auditorium, the state's largest convention center. Polly worked part-time as a private secretary. Arriving home within minutes of each other that Monday afternoon, they found their son sitting on the couch in the living room holding icecubes wrapped in a towel to his puffed cheek.

"John! What happened?" Polly asked anxiously.

John shrugged. "I was practicing on the mesa and just stumbled over my feet." Absentmindedly he tugged at his shirt-front to ease the pressure of his clothing against his chest. Recently he had been doing that often.

Jack sat down on the couch next to his son. "John," he said, "why don't you go see Doctor Follingstad?"

John sighed irritably. "Come on, Dad—just because I fell down? You know I had track physicals every year at

16

the university. They don't come any tougher than that. I'm OK. Believe me."

Jack shook his head. This time he wouldn't be put off. "That was two years ago. This is now. You've been complaining of chest pains for two weeks. You take vitamin pills, iron pills, protein pills and who knows what else, by the hundreds. Obviously they're not helping. Go get a check-up. Make sure. That's all I'm asking."

John frowned. As always the discussion of a physical examination exasperated him. But he knew his parents meant well. Why antagonize them by arguing further? He smiled. "Dad, I'm sure it's just a pulled muscle or something. I've been doing a lot of weight lifting to keep toned. But when school's out for summer, I'll get a check-up. I promise." Without waiting for a response he jumped up from the couch and looked at his watch. "Hey, I'm sorry, but I've got to run. I promised Haaland I'd play basketball tonight." He started toward the door.

"John," Polly called after him, "what about your dinner?"

"I'll get a bite downtown, Mom. See you later."

Jack and Polly looked at each other resignedly. John's promise to get a check-up when school let out in two weeks was more than he'd agreed to before. With little alternative, they accepted it as half-a-loaf.

Three blocks from home John pulled his Triumph into a service station. He had no plans to play basketball that evening with John Haaland. But he urgently needed to talk to his best friend. For despite his show of nonchalance to his parents, he was deeply worried about what had happened that afternoon. He had reasons. Reasons he'd mentioned to no one. Now, he was determined to bring his secret fears into the open.

From an outside pay phone near the station he dialed John Haaland's number. He was relieved when Haaland answered.

"Hey," Baker said, "what's on tonight?"

Haaland recognized Baker's voice at once. "I've got a date for a late flick," Haaland replied. "What's up?"

"Oh . . . nothing in particular. I just thought that if you had nothing going we could ride around and talk."

This was no ordinary call. There was something in Baker's voice Haaland hadn't heard before. Worry? It was more than that. "Look," Haaland said. "I've got a couple of hours. Are you close by?"

"Yes," Baker replied.

"Pick me up in fifteen minutes."

Haaland was standing at the curb in front of his apartment when Baker pulled up. As always when he climbed into Baker's car, Haaland swore. Standing six foot two—three inches taller than Baker—Haaland couldn't fit his lanky frame comfortably in the tiny Triumph. He made a great show of squirming around in the seat. "Why don't you junk this sardine can and get yourself a motorcycle?" Haaland complained. Haaland was a motorcycle buff.

Baker ignored the kidding, which wasn't like him at all.

They drove in silence. Haaland was worried. He'd known Baker since fifth grade. Throughout highschool and college they'd shared dreams, problems and confidences. Since their early teens, whenever pressures mounted, they'd often retreated to the mountains for a weekend with backpacks to talk out each other's problems. Now that they were both elementary-school coaches they often discussed professional matters. Haaland had seen Baker low before. But never like this. He decided to press the issue.

"All right," Haaland said, trying to keep things light

18

"let's see if I can guess. You just got a 'dear John' from Mary Ann. She'd ditching you for a sailor—worse, a football player."

Baker shot Haaland a reproachful glance.

"Bad joke, huh?" Haaland said.

With a half-smile Baker nodded. They had reached a favorite drive-in restaurant near the University of New Mexico campus. Baker pulled in and parked. They ordered Cokes. Baker sipped his silently.

Haaland tried again. "Has it got anything to do with that shiner on your cheek?"

Baker nodded. "I fell today . . . on the mesa," he said quietly, keeping his eyes on his drink.

"So?" Haaland replied. "You've fallen before. So have I. All runners do."

Baker shook his head. "Not like this, they don't. It wasn't a stumble. I . . . blacked out." He described the whole scene—the sudden loss of sight, the excruciating pain, the slow recovery of his senses, the struggle to walk. "But that's not all." He turned and looked gravely at Haaland. "John, I've got a lump, like a marble—on my balls of all damn places. And I think it's getting bigger. I'm afraid it could have something to do with the other . . . the pain in my groin today, my chest pains. Do you think it's possible?"

Haaland was shaken. No imagined scenario of what might be bothering Baker had involved anything like this. Haaland put himself on guard. He knew his friend well. It would be easy to downplay Baker's concern. Instinctively, Haaland recognized this was no time for evasions. He shook his head. "I can't answer that. And neither can you. Have you seen a doctor?"

Baker shook his head. "I promised my folks I would when school lets out for summer vaction."

19

"Summer vaction! Man, are you loco? You just said you suspect you've got a serious problem. OK. Maybe you do and maybe you don't. But in your next breath you tell me you're not going to do anything about it for two more weeks. That's plain stupid. You've got more smarts than that. Look, I want your promise you'll see a doctor first thing tomorrow."

Baker was startled by Haaland's urgency. "I know you're right," he said hesitantly.

"Then I have your promise?"

Baker looked at Haaland thoughtfully. "Yes," he said at last. "Tomorrow."

"Good," Haaland said. "Now, get me back home. I still have a date, you know."

The next morning Baker woke up feeling fine. As usual he ran in place beside his bed for several minutes. No problem. He pressed his hands firmly against his chest. It was hard, and there was no pain. He sat down on his bed, enormously relieved. Just as he'd figured all along. Yesterday was a freak occurrence—one of those episodes that never gets explained. No reason to worry about it. Then he remembered his promise to Haaland. *Well,* he thought, *no need to keep it now.*

In high spirits he showered, dressed, ate a big breakfast and went to his job at Aspen Elementary School. He'd explain to Haaland the next time they got together. His friend would understand.

All was right with the world.

Chapter 2

Wednesday morning John woke up with a sense of foreboding. It wasn't pain. It was something else. A heaviness. He moved his hand down under the covers to examine himself and withdrew it with a start. Jumping out of bed, he kicked off his pajamas and stood in front of the dresser mirror. "Good God!" he gasped. His left testicle was swollen to three times normal size.

He dressed quickly and went to the kitchen where his mother was just starting breakfast. He sat down at the small kitchen table. "Mom," he said after a moment, "I think I've got a hernia."

Polly turned from the stove and looked at her son uneasily. She started to speak. But before her words could come John held up his hands defensively. "I know, I know," he said. Without another word he stepped over to the kitchen phone and dialed the office of the Bakers' family physician, Doctor A. H. Follingstad.

Doctor Follingstad's nurse receptionist listened as John described his symptoms.

"Mr. Baker," the nurse said, "I think you should come in at once."

Characteristically, John delayed. Unwilling to miss a day at Aspen he made the appointment for two o'clock. That afternoon, forewarned, Doctor Follingstad ushered John directly into his office. The examination was quick. Then, while John dressed, Follingstad began to write on a small notepad.

"Is it a hernia, Doctor?" John asked.

Follingstad shook his head. "I don't think so. But let's make sure." He handed John the note. "Here's the name of a specialist—a urologist. I want you to go see him. I'll let him know you're coming."

John studied the note: Dr. Edward L. Johnson. The name was followed by an address. John looked up, puzzled. "When?" he asked.

"Right now," Follingstad replied.

Thirty minutes later John lay on his back on a narrow examination table, staring at a white tile ceiling. The position was humiliating. Like a woman in labor, he had his feet planted in elevated stirrups. At the end of the table, in the glare of a probe lamp, Doctor Johnson—a stranger—was examining him with acutely embarrassing thoroughness. John had never known a hernia examination like this.

Suddenly the probe lamp switched off. "All right, John," Doctor Johnson said. "You can get dressed now. When you're ready, come through that door to my office so we can talk."

At his desk Ed Johnson opened John's new patient file and began to write. The symptoms were ominous. From years of experience Johnson was almost certain he knew what lay ahead for John Baker.

A few minutes later John stepped into the office, tucking his shirt-tail into his trousers. He sat down in a comfortable leather chair at the end of the desk and sized Johnson up. Slightly shorter than John, but stockier, Johnson moved almost athletically. His dark-brown hair was conservatively crew cut. He was thirty-six years old. John had expected an older man.

Johnson put down his pen and studied his patient carefully. Only a dozen years older than John, Johnson could all too easily empathize with the younger man. "John, you have a testicular tumor. They take several forms. Exactly what type you have I can't tell at this point. But one thing is certain. The testicle must be removed at once."

Castration! John's mind reeled.

Johnson was prepared for the reaction. He shook his head. "It won't make you impotent. These things usually affect one gland. The other usually functions normally."

John breathed deeply for control. "But, I thought . . . it was something else." His voice was barely audible. "You're sure? I mean . . . it's absolutely necessary?"

Johnson nodded firmly. "It's imperative, John."

John tried to gather his jumbled thoughts. The doctor's tone was friendly, concerned, far from the professional detachment John had expected. But, an operation—on his manhood! Still hesitant, he asked, "When? Can it wait until school's out for summer?"

Johnson shook his head. The tumor had already outgrown its core blood supply and was hemorrhaging. "No, John. It can't." Johnson deliberately scanned his appointment schedule. "I'd like to book you for surgery first thing Monday morning." He looked at John for a response.

So soon, John thought desperately. *Fait accompli.* There was obviously more to this than Johnson was letting on. "Doctor, I'm a distance runner. I'm in training for the Olympics . . ."

"I know," Johnson said. "I'm a fan of yours."

John smiled, honestly grateful for this recognition, for this unexpected bond between them. Somehow it put him more at ease.

"Tell me the truth, Doctor. Will I still be able to run?"

Johnson hesitated. It was always the same. How to emphasize the seriousness of the situation without destroying hope. "I can't tell you before the operation. But there's a possibility the tumor may not be confined to your testicle."

"May not be confined? Doctor Johnson, you're talking cancer!"

"I'm sorry. But it can't be ruled out. If pathology bears out malignancy then we'll have to explore further to determine the extent of its spread. That can be done immediately, while you're still in surgery. Or in a second operation later on. We'll cross that bridge when we come to it." Johnson leaned forward on his desk and looked directly at John. "But for right now, from this moment on, you must begin preparing yourself for some possibly harsh new realities in your life."

There was a long silence. From the anguish on John's face, Johnson knew his point had finally been made. He turned back to his schedule book. Without comment, John nodded approval of the Monday morning surgery.

But something puzzled Johnson. If the tumor in John's

24

testicle was the type the symptoms indicated, it was unmistakably long-seated.

"John," Johnson inquired, "when did you first notice anything different about your testicle?"

"I've had this lump for about a week. Then, this morning, the swelling . . ."

"No. Before that. There must have been something. A smaller nodule, maybe?"

John's eyes widened. "Nodule! Oh my God. My draft physical."

"Draft physical?" Johnson repeated.

John nodded. Then he told an alarming story. In September 1966, he recounted, he had been called in by the Albuquerque Selective Service office for a preinduction physical. Several days later he received a notice that he was "medically unqualified" for military service.

"Why?" Johnson asked.

" 'Fallen arches,' they said. But I remember something else, now. During the examination the doctor told me I had a nodule on my left testicle. He asked if it bothered me. I told him I didn't even know it was there. He said it was nothing serious and not to worry about it. Honest-to-God. Even lately when I started feeling the lump I didn't connect it with that nodule. But it's the same. I know that now." He shook his head forlornly.

The tumor had been discovered over two-and-a-half years earlier—by a physician!

Ed Johnson found himself struggling to maintain his professional cool. It wouldn't do, he knew, to upset his patient unduly. But John's story was distressing. *Whether another example of impersonal, assembly-line medicine,* Johnson

25

thought, *or the ignorance of an unwary physician, the result was the same—a missed opportunity for cure.* Discovered in early nodule form, the type of tumor John obviously had was 95 percent curable. In later stages it was often terminal. Nor could John himself be blamed, Johnson knew. An alarming fact about testicular tumors was the number of men who were unaware of a lump or nodule that had obviously been on their testicles for months. Indeed, a high number of nodules were discovered by a man's wife or girlfriend, during sex, rather than by the man himself. *If only men—particularly young men—were urged to examine their scrotum regularly, as women were counseled to examine their breasts,* Johnson thought. For him the "ignored nodule" would remain the most tragic aspect of the John Baker story.

The athlete and the doctor talked for a while longer. Though up-tight, John appeared in control.

"Do you have any questions for now, John?" Johnson asked. "Anything I haven't made clear?"

John shook his head. "No questions. But maybe a favor?"

"What?"

"About the nodule—its being discovered so long ago and all. That would hurt my parents too much. I don't want them to know about it now."

"I understand. I won't mention it." Johnson rose and stepped around his desk. "If you have any questions, any problems at all, call me—night or day."

As John would learn, it was no idle offer.

Johnson's urgency had not escaped John. A half-hour later he was ransacking the book stacks in the University of New Mexico Medical School Library. After a short search he found what he was looking for—a textbook on urological cancers. He sat at a near-by table and read and reread the chapters on testicular tumors. Before long he knew more than he cared to know. He closed the book grimly. The abomination in his groin was death.

Outside the library he spotted a pay phone. Nervously, he dialed his father's office. Jack wasn't in. "No," the secretary replied, "I don't know where to reach him."

Frustrated, John slammed the phone back on the hook. His car was at the curb just across the campus mall. He slid behind the wheel and sat there without starting the engine. On the mall a group of students stood laughing, gossiping, holding hands. They weren't much younger than he. Suddenly, he wanted to scream at them, to strike out at their innocence. He gripped the wheel until his knuckles turned white. "Get hold," he muttered to himself. "You can't go home like this."

Home. His stomach churned. How do you tell your parents you're dying?

Jack and Polly had learned long before not to hold dinner for their busy son. They had already started to eat when his car pulled into the driveway. Jack readied his customary barb about latecomers getting leftovers, but one glance at his son's face stopped him.

John walked over to the kitchen table and sat down. "Follingstad sent me to a specialist. A urologist."

"A urologist?" Jack repeated, puzzled.

John nodded. He told them about Doctor Johnson's diagnosis. "I'm scheduled for surgery Monday morning."

This is not real, Polly thought. *I must say something, make some clever remark to bring us all back to reality.*

27

But it was Jack who spoke first. "John, lots of people have tumors removed without any problem at all. These things are usually benign. You'll see."

Polly agreed at once. "Your father's right." She paused. "I wonder if we should call Bob and Jill, and Mary Ann?" Bob and Jill, John's younger brother and sister, lived out of town. So did his fiancée, Mary Ann Allison.

John shook his head. "This is an exploratory operation, Mom. I'll call everybody when I find out what's what and how long it's going to take me to beat this thing."

Polly reached across the table and took her son's hand. "It's going to be all right, John. You caught it early. That's the important thing."

John patted his mother's hand. "Sure. It's going to be OK." He got up and went to his room and closed the door. Against the far wall beneath the window stood a large ranch-oak bookcase. There were no books in it. Instead, the shelves were crowded with trophies. There were statues and cups—gold, silver and bronze—of varying sizes. He moved his desk chair to the bookcase and sat down. This was his private world, the archive of the most cherished achievements of his lifetime. *A very short lifetime!* he thought bitterly.

He ran his hand fondly over the trophies. It came to rest on the smallest one, perched in a prominent position on the top shelf. It depicted a runner in full pace. He lifted the tiny statue and read the inscription etched on its base:

JOHN BAKER
CROSS-COUNTRY CHAMPION
MANZANO–HIGHLAND DUAL MEET
SEPTEMBER 1960

* * *

He smiled. The first trophy he'd ever won. He'd fooled them all. He'd even fooled himself.

As he thought back, it didn't seem so long ago. . . .

Chapter 3

Many residents of Albuquerque's Northeast Heights remember the day the Baker family moved into the neighborhood. It would be a hard day to forget, for the Bakers arrived "on camera."

In the 1940s Jack Baker's name was a household word in
millions of homes coast-to-coast. Radio and television fans
of the era will remember him as the thickset, ruddy-faced
impresario of *Don McNeil's Breakfast Club*, a popular variety show broadcast from Chicago. He starred for McNeil
for eight years. Then, in 1943, following his marriage to one
of his most ardent fans, twenty-year-old, raven-haired Polly Willoughby, from Ben Wheeler, Texas, he switched
from performing to station management in the rapidly expanding field of television.

For the next eleven years Jack and Polly traveled extensively while Jack managed TV stations in Arkansas, Mis-

31

souri, Illinois, Tennessee and Wisconsin. On June 29, 1944, in Springfield, Missouri, their first child, John, was born. For Jack it was a day for double celebration. It was his thirty-sixth birthday.

Two years later, in Nashville, on September 7, 1946, a second son, Robert, was born. Then, on January 16, 1948, in Memphis, the birth of a daughter, Jill, completed the Baker family.

In 1953, with growing children, Jack and Polly became concerned about the effect of their rootless lives on the family. That spring Jack was contracted to launch and manage a new station, KOAT–TV(ABC), in Albuquerque. He fell headlong in love with the city. The clear mountain air and unlimited elbow room were ideal for raising a family. A week later he moved his family from Wisconsin to New Mexico. settled them in a rental apartment, and started searching for a permanent home.

In June a prominent building contractor visited Jack at his office. The contractor was starting a new housing development and wanted publicity. Jack was still looking for a house, and the contractor agreed to build Jack a house at cost in exchange for Jack's personal appearances in commericals for the company. For the next eight weeks Channel 7 viewers were treated to a brick-by-brick account of the construction of "The House That Jack Built."

On August 29, 1954, while television cameras broadcast the scene live, Jack, Polly, John, Robert and Jill walked through streaming banners into their new house at 1700 Kentucky Street, Northeast. The Bakers were home at last.

From his first days in Albuquerque, ten-year-old John learned that his past uprooting held an unexpected advantage. His knowledge of strange places and practices, coupled with his outgoing personality, made him an instant hit with his new pals. Though skinny and inches shorter than most of them, it was still John who took the lead in organizing activities, assigning roles and settling disputes. And he knew some exciting new games. One was "Tug."

"Tug" was played at evening just after dusk, when lengthening shadows made visibility poor. On opposite sides of Kentucky Street, John and a companion would crouch behind shrubs and await an oncoming car. Just as the driver reached their hiding places both boys would leap up, pretend to grasp opposite ends of an imaginary rope, and loudly yell, "TUG!"

"Seeing" the threatening barrier, motorists would screech to a jolting halt. Then, as angry curses filled the air, the culprits would flee to safety, laughing all the way. One evening John's partner was his eight-year-old brother, Robert. But this night the motorist didn't simply sit and curse. He leaped from his car and gave chase. Robert escaped, but John was caught.

Ten minutes later the irate motorist, John in tow, stood on the Bakers' porch telling Jack what had happened. Punishment was swift. After a stern lecture, John was assigned to do all the household chores—cleaning, dusting, dishwashing, garbage carryout—for one week.

Robert was remorseful. "I gotta tell Dad," he whispered down from his upper bunk that night in the room he shared with John.

"No way!" John replied. "You escaped. Now keep quiet."

Reluctantly, Robert agreed. But secretly, all that week, he helped John do the chores.

At the end of the week Jack took John aside. "I hope,

33

young man," Jack said, "that all this has taught you a lesson."

"It sure has," John agreed. "I gotta learn to run faster."

The next morning John called his friends to come over and bring rakes, hoes and shovels. When they arrived he assembled them at the rear of his house where the mesa lay in open range. Just behind his back fence he and his friends spent the day scraping away tumbleweeds, cacti and sagebrush, until they had cleared an area suitable for a ball diamond. That evening, in a rousing game of softball, umpired by his father, John began to train himself to run faster.

In September the Baker children entered nearby Mark Twain Elementary School. John was in the fifth grade. Unlike Robert, who approached his studies indifferently but still made high marks, John had to struggle for good grades. But determination was already one of his traits. At the first PTA meeting that year his teacher took Polly aside. "Mrs. Baker," she asked, a bit apprehensively, "do you and your husband . . . well . . . demand perfection in your children?"

Puzzled, Polly asked for an explanation.

"John is so intense," she said. "He gets upset with himself when he can't grasp a lesson right off. He sometimes works through recess."

Polly laughed. "Next year you'll get Robert in your class. You'll see then that John's doggedness is his own doing, not a Baker trait."

The following year she reminded Polly of their talk. "I see what you meant," the teacher said.

On the first day of school a gangly, handsome, tow-headed boy walked up to John on the playground and looked down on him from a two-inch advantage in height. "You John Baker?" the tow-head demanded.

"Yeah."

The tow-head nodded toward some boys who stood with him. "We hear you're supposed to have a hot-shot ball team over on Kentucky Street."

"That's twice you're right," John replied.

"My name's John Haaland. I say we've got a better team. Wanta find out, this afternoon—your field?"

"We'll be waiting," Baker said.

At six-o'clock that evening, with the score tied 20-to-20 in the fourteenth inning, two bone-weary teams decided to call it a draw. Exhausted, the team captains, Baker and Haaland, dropped to the ground and sat back against the Bakers' rear fence. The aroma of the evening meal wafted toward them.

"Hungry?" Baker asked.

"You kidding!" Haaland exclaimed. "I could eat a coyote."

"All we got's chicken."

"That'll do."

That evening John Baker and John Haaland shared the first of many meals they would eat over the years at each other's homes. It was the beginning of a lasting friendship.

By the time he entered highschool John had become a competent outfielder, and he made the freshman team. Then, in his sophomore year, his sports career almost came to an end. That year, with a rapidly expanding student population, the Albuquerque school districts were realigned. While his new highschool was under construction, John was temporarily assigned to another district. Within weeks his morale plummeted, and his grades began to drop. One afternoon, Jack took him aside and asked for an explanation. After some hesitation, John said, "Dad, I've got a problem at school."

35

"Tell me about it," Jack said.

John explained. At the end of the first week, when he hadn't reported for baseball practice, he'd been called to a coach's office. The coach had demanded to know why John hadn't come out for practice.

"I was thinking about waiting for track," John had replied.

"Track?" the coach had retorted. "Are you kidding? A scrawny kid like you? You wouldn't stand a chance. Besides, on my campus you play what I say you play." He pointed a finger at John's face. "And I say you'll be at ball practice this afternoon. Hear?"

Throughout John's story, Jack's anger had mounted. "And?" he asked.

"I didn't go," John said. "And I'm not going. But now the coach is picking on me. He puts me down in class and everywhere."

Jack looked at his watch. Ball practice would still be going on at the school. Without another word he left the house, got into his car and drove away. When he returned a half-hour later, John was sitting at the kitchen table with Polly. "There won't by any more picking on you at school, John," Jack said firmly. "I can promise you that." Though Jack never again mentioned the incident, or what he'd said to the coach, the pressure on John ceased. His pride in his father, always high, soared. Moreover, he'd learned a lesson about the negative side of coaching that he'd never forget.

He stayed away from school sports for the remainder of that year. Then, in his junior year, he initiated a turn-of-events that changed the course of his life.

In 1960, along with most of his chums, John was transferred to newly opened Manzano High School. He was sixteen. Eager to build a first-rate track team from the beginning, Manzano's coach, Bill Wolffarth, had his eye on a promising young athlete—John Haaland. But his overtures to Haaland fell on deaf ears.

One afternoon Baker went to Wolffarth's office. "Coach, I hear you've been trying to recruit Haaland?" Baker commented.

"Trying is about all," Wolffarth admitted.

John's brown eyes flashed merrily. "I'll make you a deal. Let me join the track team and I'll get Haaland to join too."

Wolffarth chuckled. Baker a runner? He looked at the boy fondly. He liked him, had known him ever since grade school. But Baker was too short-legged, too uncoordinated for track. Still, he *was* Haaland's best friend.

"You really think you can deliver on that deal, old buddy?"

"I know I can," John replied.

Wolffarth thought for a long moment. The kid had spunk. "Tell you what," Wolffarth said. "You have Haaland here at two-thirty tomorrow. Both of you dressed out. And you've got a deal."

John flashed a winning smile. "We'll be here."

When John left, Wolffarth shook his head. He had no hopes for the boy as a runner. It was the most fortunate misjudgment of his career.

The first meet that fall was a 1.7-mile cross-country race through the foothills of the Sandia Mountains just east of Albuquerque. Under a bright sky a crowd of two hundred fans clustered around the starting line to watch twelve runners limber up. Most eyes were focused on Highland High

37

School's reigning state champion miler, Lloyd Goff. Speculation centered on how closely Manzano's new hope, John Haaland, could trail the champion. No one paid attention to another Manzano entry: number 33; height 5 feet 6 inches; weight, 135 pounds; previous entries, none; name—John Baker.

At the crack of the gun the runners kicked off, pacing themselves slowly in the mile-high mountain air. The field lined up as predicted. Goff set the pace with Haaland following closely. At the end of four minutes the runners disappeared behind a low hill just inside the far turn of the flag-marked course. The spectators switched their gaze to where the runners would emerge from behind the hill. A minute passed. Two. Then a lone figure appeared.

Kneeling near the finish line, squinting against the sun, Bill Wolffarth nudged an assistant. "Well, here comes Goff." Wolffarth raised his binoculars. With an ear-splitting yelp he jumped straight up in the air. "That's not Goff," he screamed. "That's Baker!"

Pounding toward the homestretch, John grinned and glanced back over his shoulder.

"Don't look back, boy!" Wolffarth shouted. "Run! Run!"

Leaving a field of surprised runners behind, John crossed the finish line in 8:30.5. He had not only scored an upset, he had set a new meet record. The crowd cheered wildly.

What had happened on the far side of that hill? Later that evening John told his family.

Halfway through the race, with things going as expected, he had asked himself: *Is this my best?* He didn't know. Resolutely, he fixed his eye on the back number of the front runner. He closed his mind to everything else. Only one thing mattered: catch and pass that number—that runner. A new energy surged through his body. It was almost hypnotic. One by one he passed the front runners, then took a commanding lead. Forcing himself to ignore the fatigue tearing at his muscles, he maintained his furious pace until he crossed the finish line and collapsed in exhaustion. He was to repeat that pattern many times.

Elated at finding this unexpected talent, Wolffarth tried John in other events: cross-country, the mile, the medley relay. The result was always the same. On the track the modest fun-loving teenager became a relentless competitor. Doubts dispelled, Wolffarth rebuilt his team around Manzano's new star—John Baker.

One day an assistant coach criticized John's style. "His form is terrible. He tilts his face up like he's looking for rain. Look how he throws that right leg."

"True," Wolffarth replied. He fixed his assistant with a no-nonsense stare. "But you don't change feed on a winning horse."

To sportswriters who were just beginning to notice John, Wolffarth put it differently: "It doesn't come easy to Baker. He's a heart runner. A triumph of determination over style."

By the end of his first year in competitive track, John had broken six state records.

In his senior year John carried the Manzano purple-and-gray to victory after victory in individual wins as records continued to fall to his free-style onslaught. By spring of 1962, sportswriters were predicting he would complete the season undefeated.

Then came the last meet of the year.

New Mexico's finest highschool runners converged on

Wm. J. Buchanan

Albuquerque's University Stadium that afternoon of May 12, 1962, for the fiftieth Annual State Championship Track and Field Meet. Conditions were not ideal. The temperature in the mile-high city was forty-one degrees. A steady north wind gusted at time to forty miles-per-hour. Worst of all, swirling clouds of dust and sand, whipped up from the surrounding desert, plagued the runners, clogging their throats and irritating their eyes.

Midway in the meet Bill Wolffarth pondered tactics. He knew Manzano was in trouble. The coveted first-, second- and third-place team positions had already been won on points by older schools with long-established sports programs. But to finish in the top five against such experienced competition would be a respectable prize for Manzano. To win fifth place Manzano had to take the next race—the medley relay. It was Manzano's weakest event.

The medley relay was a one-mile race between four-man teams. Each starting runner had to race 220 yards (one-half lap of a standard outdoor track), then pass a baton to the second runner on his team who would also race 220 yards. The third runner would race one full lap, 440 yards. The anchor man would lap the track twice, carrying the baton a distance equaling that covered by his teammates combined, 880 yards—one-half mile.

Wolffarth knew Manzano's first three runners were outclassed. The race depended on the anchor man—John Baker. But already that afternoon John had won the mile championship race. He was undefeated for the season. Would it be fair to risk his flawless record in a second grueling race for a questionable team win? Knowing that John would insist on staying in the race, Wolffarth resisted the impulse to make a substitution.

40

Within minutes after the gun Wolffarth regretted his decision. As he feared, Manzano's first two runners were no match for their opponents. Nor could the third, buffeted by a blinding sandstorm, make up the deficit. By the time the baton was passed to John the anchor men of the opposing teams were already nearing the first turn, almost a hundred yards ahead.

High in the stands one burly spectator, rooting for another team, yelled, "Looks like that prima donna Baker isn't going to win 'em all this year after all!"

But John was tearing along. On the far turn, in the midst of his second lap, he kicked into his final sprint, 220 yards from the finish line. With each stride he gained on the front runners. Could he maintain maximum effort for such distance? The spectators rose to their feet. Entering the final turn John passed one, then another of the lead runners. He was now second. The crowd roared. Ignoring the forty-mile-per-hour headwind sandblasting his face and body, John held his sprint. With less than fifty yards to go he closed fast on the front man.

In the stands, the man who had loudly predicted John's defeat felt something strike him on the shoulder. He turned to see an attractive brunette directly behind him flailing away at his back with her fists while she screamed at the top of her lungs, "GO, JOHN! GO!" At that instant, on the track below, John crossed the finish line, a winner by inches.

When the crowd's frenzy abated, the brunette grasped the astonished man's hand and apologized profusely. "You see," a beaming Polly Baker explained, "I'm that prima donna's mother."

It was a fantastic finale to an improbable highschool

sports career. By now a prime attraction to sportswriters throughout the Southwest, John was touted as "the finest miler ever developed in New Mexico." He was not yet eighteen.

With scholarship bids from Texas Western, Arizona State, University of Arizona, the University of Oklahoma and six other colleges John chose to remain at home. He accepted an athletic scholarship to the University of New Mexico in Albuquerque.

On the first day of practice he was called to the office of Lobo track coach Hugh Hackett. A husky man, sporting an athletic crew cut and built more like a football player than a track man, Hackett had, by the fall of 1962, forged the New Mexico Lobos into a formidable power. He'd watched John's progress for two years and was impressed more by his spirit and determination than by his style. Yet, he sensed a potential for greatness in John.

"John," Hackett said during that first training meeting, in his softspoken voice, "you've had an outstanding high-school career. But you're running in a league now where everyone is outstanding. You must not forget that for a single moment while you're a Lobo."

John began a spartan routine. Each morning at dawn, spray can in hand to ward off pesky dogs, he ran through city streets, parks and golf courses—twenty-five miles a day—in addition to the regular varsity workouts.

The rigorous training told. Soon, in Phoenix, Tulsa, Denver, Lubbock, Salt Lake City, wherever the Lobos competed, their fans gloried in the exploits of "Upset John" Baker, who consistently picked off top-rated runners throughout the Western Athletic Conference.

Despite his growing fame, John's carefree nature hadn't

42

changed. One winter evening, after a successful meet at the Air Force Academy in Colorado Springs, he was riding home with John Haaland, also a Lobo runner. Haaland was driving. As they topped out at 7,834-foot-high Raton Pass, on the Colorado-New Mexico border, they spotted a white station wagon ahead.

"Hey," Baker said. "That's Hackett and some of the guys. Let's give 'em the old salute."

"Why not?" Haaland replied. He speeded up.

As they drew alongside the station wagon Baker jumped up on the front seat, dropped his pants and shorts, and stuck his bare behind out the window.

"Ohmygawd!" Haaland exclaimed suddenly. He floor-boarded the accelerator.

The sudden acceleration thrust Baker further out the window. Struggling to hold on, he tried to pull himself back inside the car, but couldn't. "Damn it, John! Slow down," he cried. "My ass is freezing!"

"I can't," Haaland replied. "That's not the guys. It's a bunch of faculty wives!"

For several minutes a carload of startled women—all wives of Baker's professors—watched wide-eyed as Baker's bare buttocks, whipped by an icy wind, receded into the night.

By 1963 Jack had left his pressure-cooker job in television for a less hectic position as manager of Albuquerque's Civic Auditorium. Polly, too, had sought a change. An accomplished guitarist and folk-singer, she had long entertained at her church, hospitals, schools and senior-citizen clubs. But with her children grown she found her usual hobbies weren't enough. So she went to work as a private secretary to the manager of the Bendix Corporation in Albuquerque. But despite their jobs, and Robert's and Jill's schooling, the Bakers remained John's most devoted fans. The family had a standing rule: whenever John ran in a meet within five hundred miles of Albuquerque, one or all of them would be there to root for him. Though it often meant late starts and all-night drives to arrive in time for the opening gun, the rule was never violated.

For as long as he could remember, Robert Baker had idolized his brother. So, when he entered highschool, Robert also went out for track. Dark-skinned, and as tall as John, but heavier built, Robert never achieved his brother's star status. But he did become a fine miler.

One day in 1964, Robert, eighteen, and John, twenty, entered back-to-back mile races in an indoor exhibition in Albuquerque.

Robert's race was first. In the homestretch he developed leg cramps, finished last, and fell to the track side exhausted. John ran to his side, just as the next event was announced. John didn't move. The announcer called for "John Baker" to report to the starting line. Still, John didn't move. The spectators watched in admiration as John tended his fallen brother, seemingly massaging his legs. What the spectators didn't know was that the Baker brothers had one pair of indoor track shoes between them. And Robert's cramped toes had furled, locking the shoes tightly to his feet. As the loudspeaker blared his name, John tugged frantically at the shoes. "For God's sake, Bob," he said, "straighten your toes!" With a violent yank, he pulled the shoes free, laced them to his feet, rushed to the starting line and took his crouch, just as the gun roared.

He won the race.

*   *   *

At fifteen, Jill had developed into a petite beauty with auburn hair and flashing dark eyes. Her looks and personality drew a steady parade of boys to the Baker home. None escaped John's critical eye. When a suitor appeared who didn't measure up to his standards, a brother-sister conference, late at night at the kitchen table, was a certainty. She didn't always take John's advice, but she never resented his caring.

One morning at track practice John asked Coach Hackett if he could be excused, promising to make up the training the next day.

"Why?" Hackett asked.

John explained his reason. Hackett chuckled and let him go.

John hurried home. As planned, Jill was waiting for him. Together they went to Manzano. It was Jill's first day of highschool.

For the rest of that morning he accompanied Jill to her classes, introduced her to teachers and walked at her side around the campus. As he knew it would be, his appearance at the school was big news. And the implication was clear. This lovely new girl at Manzano was John Baker's sister, and everybody, especially the boys, had better keep it in mind.

In spite of John's growing string of victories, a repeated and valid criticism of him was that he ran "only to win"—meaning that he raced the competition, not the clock. One result was that runners with better times tended to dismiss him as no threat. Often to their chagrin. One incident came to be known in track circles as "The Race That Crumbled Troy."

45

In the spring of 1965 the most highly regarded track team in the nation belonged to the University of Southern California. Boasting a twenty-year record of 126 victories and only two losses, the Trojans descended on Albuquerque that April for a dual meet. Sportswriters predicted doom for the Lobos. The mile, they said, would fall to USC's "Big Three"—Chris Johnson, Doug Calhoun and Bruce Bess, in that order.

At 2:30 A.M. Saturday, April 3, the day of the meet, Polly was awakened by a steady rasping noise coming from the kitchen. She recognized the sound at once. But at 2:30 in the morning! She got up to investigate. Seated at the kitchen table, track shoes in hand, John was filing his spikes. "I can't sleep," he said. "I might as well get ready for the race."

Polly had never seen her son so wrought-up. All over the floor, wadded in balls, were the sportspages from papers predicting the Trojans would run the Lobos into the ground. She went to the cupboard, took down two cups and put on a pot of tea. Till morning she sat up with her son.

At the opening gun of the mile event that afternoon, six-thousand fans in Albuquerque's University Stadium watched with surprise as John led the field for one full lap. Then, he waved at the press box, flashed a grin, and eased back into fourth place where the sportswriters had predicted he would be from the start.

It was a master psych-out. Calhoun and Bess moved into the forfeited lead. Johnson held back.

In the far turn of the third lap, with Bess and Calhoun still ahead, John and Johnson moved for the lead at the same moment—and collided. Pushed to one side, John fought to keep his feet. Less jostled, Johnson took the lead.

46

Regaining his stride, but with precious seconds lost, John decided to kick into his final sprint, with 300 yards to go. Astonished, the fans rose cheering. Bess and Calhoun fell behind. On the final turn it was Johnson and John, neck and neck. Johnson was hanging on, but the pace proved too much. Slowly, John inched ahead. Grinning, he raised his hands above his head in a V-for-victory and broke the tape—a winner by three seconds!

Inspired by John's dramatic triumph the Lobos swept every following event, handing the demoralized Trojans their third-worst defeat in sixty-five years. To newsmen who gathered around John at the meet's end, a happy Hugh Hackett said, "Baker's never run a four-minute mile. But he's beaten more four-minute milers than you can count."

On April 4, 1965, the photo of John's beaming, arm-waving victory over Troy was front-page news. It was the capstone of his racing career.

On graduation John considered his prospects as a runner. Four times he'd captured the Western Athletic Conference mile and cross-country titles. He had defeated thirty-nine "name" runners, including NCAA Champion Chris Johnson, Australian Champion John Lawler, Colorado University's Bob Griffith, Brigham Young University's Dick Kremzer, Canadian National Champion Dave Wrighton, and, in what John considered his most important upset, Olympic Gold Medalist Robert Schul. Was he good enough for the Olympics?

On June 23, 1967, he wrote Robert Schul.

Having achieved national prominence with a string of record-breaking wins in the mid-1960s, Bob Schul had captured the three-mile National Championship, the five-thou-

47

sand-meter National Championship, and the two-mile world record. Then, on Sunday, October 3, 1964, racing through a blinding, bone-chilling rainstorm, he had captured the five-thousand-meter Gold Medal for the United States in the Olympic Games in Tokyo.

In 1967, as Sports Director of the Athens Athletic Club in Oakland, California, Bob Schul was training selected runners he believed had merit. Schul remembered the scrappy Lobo miler well. He replied to John's letter at once. He'd be happy to accept him as a trainee.

Schul quickly detected flaws in John's style. Foot-plant, knee-lift, arm-carry, push-off—all were awkward. One by one over the next year, Schul corrected John's ingrained bad habits. Just as important, for the first time John learned to race the clock.

It was also in California that summer of 1967 that John met Mary Ann Allison.

Monday morning each week an Athens Athletic Club staffer hand-carried weekend receipts to a nearby bank for deposit. Pressed to perform the chore one morning, John was soon volunteering. His deposit trips took longer and longer. One morning, undetected, a friend followed him. At a teller's window he was slowly, painstakingly, transacting business with an attentive young woman who was obviously enjoying the prolonged visit.

Later that morning John returned to the club and handed the office manager the deposit slip. "Thanks, John," the manager said. "Oh, by the way. Good news. I've found someone to make the deposits from now on."

John's jaw dropped.

Unable to contain himself, the manager began to laugh at John's dismay. Suddenly, John was surrounded by friends who joined in the laughter. His secret was out. He blushed.

"Just one more deposit," he pleaded, "and I'll ask her for a date."

Ask her he did.

Small, remarkably pretty with soft brown hair and hazel eyes, and possessing a refreshing sense of humor, 23-year-old Mary Ann was a perfect match for John. On their first date, a picnic at Alameda Beach, they quickly discovered their mutual interest in hiking, swimming, jogging, soft music and foreign movies.

During the few days off from training that John allowed himself, other dates followed. They went to the beaches, the mountains, and saw the sights around San Francisco. By the end of that summer, as the relationship blossomed and endured, their friends recognized that the star runner who used to enjoy playing the field, and the equally popular Mary Ann, were deeply in love.

During Christmas vacation John brought Mary Ann to Albuquerque to meet his family. It was a first meeting none of them would forget.

Fond of surprises, John arranged a flight that arrived in Albuquerque a day earlier than they were expected. They took a taxi from the airport. Arriving at his home in the late afternoon, they found the house empty. John let them in with his key and settled in the den to await the arrival of his parents.

As they sat waiting, John's eye fell on a six-foot-long replica of a Zulu spear he had made at YMCA camp during his early teens. Draped over the spear was an authentic bone-and-boar's-tooth necklace he'd strung at the same time. Grinning devilishly, he jumped up and grabbed the spear. "Go to the kitchen window and watch," he told a puzzled Mary Ann. "But keep quiet, hear?"

It was dusk when Polly got home. Other houses up and

49

down Kentucky Street were already lighted. But the Baker home was dark. As she made her way up the walk toward the front porch Polly stopped abruptly. A low, guttural cry came from somewhere in the darkness. Polly looked around quickly. Deciding her ears must have been playing tricks on her, she started again for the house. Suddenly, from somewhere above, came a louder cry, BOOGA BOO-GA KIMBAY-EE-E-E!''

Her heart in her throat, Polly wheeled in her tracks just in time to see a near-naked, loin-clothed savage, wearing a barbaric bone necklace and brandishing a long spear, leap down from the large front-yard elm tree and land directly in front of her. Just as she opened her mouth to scream, the "savage" embraced her, planted a kiss on her cheek and said, "Hi, Mom! Come on in and meet my fiancée."

Robert had enlisted in the Air Force and was in Goose Bay, Canada, that Christmas, but the rest of the Bakers took to Mary Ann with enthusiasm, and she to them.

"Mom, Dad," John told his parents that first evening at dinner. "I hope you're not offended. But I've already talked to Reverend Hawk about Mary Ann and me."

The Bakers beamed. "We're not offended, John," Jack replied. Like all popular athletes, John had had scores of girlfriends. But this time, Jack and Polly recognized joyfully, their son was deeply committed.

Throughout that happy Christmas season Mary Ann fitted in with the Baker clan, John's hometown friends, and his favorite haunts as if she had been preparing for this involvement all her life. Jill was particularly pleased. Near the same age, exactly the same size and with remarkably similar personalities, the two hit it off from the beginning. On the weekend before Christmas, Jill accompanied John

50

and Mary Ann to El Paso. They checked into the Holiday Inn and walked across the bridge spanning the Rio Grande to the bustling border city of Juarez. Delighted with the inexpensive shops, the two girls spent the day excitedly buying presents for friends, family and themselves. Burdened with packages, John at last called time out. They returned to their motel. In the room they shared, Jill and Mary Ann tried on blouses, jeans, boots and jackets, their own purchases and each other's. Exhausted at last, they fell across the bed, laughing at the chaos of strewn-about clothes. "Oh, Mary Ann," Jill said. "You're going to be a perfect sister."

The holidays at an end, John and Mary Ann said goodbye to his family at the airport. As they walked toward the loading ramp, John put his arm around Mary Ann. "Don't worry," he called back to his familiy. "Pretty soon I'll be bringing her back to stay."

In February 1968, after eight months of arduous training under Bob Schul's professional eye, John ran the mile in the National AAU Indoor Track Meet in Oakland in 4:03. Schul hurried to the dressing room to congratulate his protégé. There was no doubt in his mind now that John would soon break the four-minute mile.

John was sitting on a bench, leaning against a locker. He was pale and seemed drained of vitality. Schul was disturbed. Lately, John had been taking longer and longer to recuperate after a race. Schul sat down on the bench. "Are you all right, John?" he asked.

John nodded. "Just pooped."

"John," Schul said, "I've trained two men this year who are definitely Olympic caliber. You're one. You're every

51

bit as good as I was at your age, maybe better. But you're only twenty-three. Distance runners peak later than that. I'm convinced that if you keep training you're well on your way to your dream in 1972.''

It was one of the happiest moments of John's life.

By the beginning of summer there was nothing more for John to learn from Schul. It was time to go home. Late one evening in June, as they had on countless evenings before, John and Mary Ann strolled hand-in-hand along Alameda Beach on San Francisco Bay.

Alone by the water's edge they sat down on a low rock jetty that jutted out into the bay. During the stroll from the car John had been strangely quiet. He emptied the sand out of his loafers. At last he said, ''I'm not going to accept any of the college coaching offers, Mary Ann.'' He looked at her expectantly. ''I've decided to take the coaching job at Aspen Elementary School in Albuquerque.''

''That's wonderful, John. I figured you would all along.''

''It's really ideal. I've always wanted to coach young children—not college level.''

''I know.''

''There's so much more you can do for kids. Besides, there'll be plenty of time for me to keep up my training for the Olympics.'' He hesitated a moment. ''Mom and Dad say we can have my room at home if we want to get married right away, instead of waiting.''

It was unexpected. Mary Ann looked at him, puzzled. ''What do you want me to say, John?''

John jumped up, moved in front of Mary Ann and cupped her face in his hands. ''I *want* you to say, 'Yippee! Horray! Let's tie the knot.''' They both laughed. He dropped his hands to her shoulder. ''But I know that's not right for us, and I think you know it too. I don't want us to have to sponge off our parents—yours or mine. I want us to be able to pay our own way, have our own place. It's going to take a while. But with my job at Aspen and yours at the bank we should be able to save enough to get married next summer and start out independent. What do you think?"

"I think that's about as long as I'm going to let you put me off, John Baker—that's what I think."

They decided to marry in the summer of 1969. Until then they would write often and visit each other whenever they could. Mary Ann put her arms around John's waist and pulled him to her. "John, I'm so happy. I love you so much."

"I love you too, Mary Ann."

She looked up into his eyes. "Let's go back to the car."

They stalled their bittersweet goodbye until dawn.

In September 1968 John began his teaching and coaching career. On his playing fields at Aspen there were no "stars." Criticism for lack of ability was banned. Earnest tryers were praised as highly as winners. John was extraordinarily patient and understanding with children—his only demand was that each child do his or her best.

An inveterate chart maker, he separated his students into groups based on athletic ability. He arrived at a handicap for each child, on any team, in any sport. Soon, every child at Aspen physically capable was competing with his peers on an almost equal basis. John's fairness, plus his obvious concern for their welfare, triggered an instinctive response from the kids. Youthful grievances were brought first to Coach Baker. Real or fancied, each was treated as if at the moment it was the most important matter in the world.

53

Veta Mercer, the principal of Aspen Elementary, was delighted. A tall, attractive brunette, with a brilliant smile and an easygoing administrative manner, she had definite ideas about a coach's role in elementary schools. With so few men teachers in the early grades it was imperative, she felt, that young students be exposed to a male influence that was understanding but self-assured. At first she worried about John's "superjock" image. But as time passed she dismissed her concern. Seeing his effect on the children she began referring students whom other teachers considered "problems" to him. The results were remarkable. Underachievers took on catch-up work simply because "Coach asked." By the end of that first fall semester Mrs. Mercer was convinced that in John Baker she was witnessing a great teacher in the making.

During Christmas vacation John flew to California to spend five days with Mary Ann as a guest in her parents' home. In April 1969, during Easter, Mary Ann returned the visit. On Easter morning she presented Jack and Polly with a crystal salad bowl and a pair of sterling silver salad tongs. As he served himself from the bowl that evening, John feigned a sulk. "You didn't bring me anything, did you?"

"Sure," Mary Ann retorted, "the best present of all— me."

They all laughed.

By the end of spring, 1969, now with hundreds of "his kids" to cheer him on, John bore down hard on the four-minute mile. Slowly, he cut away the stubborn fractions of seconds. Munich and 1972 beckoned. It was the best of all worlds.

Until that May morning on the mesa when he blacked out and fell.

*   *   *

Reverie ended, John gently placed the little silver trophy back on top of the bookcase. Now he understood why the four-minute mile had proved so elusive, and why he had experienced the overlong recovery times after workouts. All through his final year at the university, and during the vigorous training meets in California, his real opponent had been not another runner, not even time, but cancer.

He looked at his watch. It was nine-thirty. *Had he eaten?* he wondered. *No matter. He wasn't hungry.* He went to his desk, opened the bottom drawer and picked up a small plastic bottle. It contained two sleeping pills. He undressed, climbed into bed and swallowed the pills without water, Shivering involuntarily, he curled into a fetal ball. Then, unable to control himself, he began to cry. He buried his face in the pillow. Then a dark thought hit him, which he tried to erase from his mind, but couldn't. He thought of the two pills he'd just taken.

He wished he had a hundred.

Chapter 4

Monday, June 2, 1969, at Presbyterian Hospital, Doctor Johnson removed John's tumorous left testicle. Examination of the badly deformed gland told him his diagnosis was sadly correct. Minutes later pathology confirmed it. The tumor was malignant.

Johnson sutured the wound quickly, then gave John an injection that would be the first of many chemotherapy treatments. The entire operation took less than thirty minutes.

At John's request Johnson waited to brief him when he revived. When the recovery room nurse reported he was awake, Johnson went in and checked his patient's vital signs. "How do you feel, John?"

"OK, I guess. I don't hurt any."

Johnson drew the blanket back over John. He was alert

enough to understand. "John, I'm sorry. The tumor was malignant."

Though he had tried to steel himself for this moment, John stared blankly at Johnson, not responding.

Johnson continued. "It's called embryonal cell carcinoma. It originates in disease-prone cells that are probably present, but dormant, from birth. Suddenly, something triggers them into malignant growth."

John swallowed hard. "Then it means another operation?"

Johnson nodded. "Your other symptoms—the chest pains, the breast sensitivity—suggest the tumor has spread. I can't be certain how far without a full exploratory."

John recoiled at the term. "You mean you want to cut me open . . . right down the middle." His voice was tense.

"We must remove any affected nodes, John."

John turned his eyes to the ceiling. The muscles of his jaws contracted spasmodically. "When?"

"As soon as your system will tolerate it. Two weeks at most."

"Then what?"

"Then we fight," Johnson said. "We use radiation, chemotherapy, every weapon at our disposal."

"For how long, Doctor?" John asked pointedly. "Just how long do we fight?"

His real question was obvious.

"I can't honestly say," Johnson replied. "It depends on many things. What we find in the next operation; how you respond to treatment; *your cooperation.*" He emphasized the last factor. "But I promise you this. After the operation I'll give you as definite a prognosis as I can."

After a long pause, John nodded.

Johnson put his hand on John's shoulder. "You'll be going back to your room soon. Your parents are waiting to see you. I think I should brief them first."

Silently, John nodded again.

Jack and Polly were waiting in the lounge just off surgery. Johnson asked them to join him in a private office. Without being obvious he scrutinized them. The father was on edge, but in control. The mother—more composed, certainly. Johnson decided both of them could tolerate the truth. "The tumor was malignant," he said. "John's doing fine now. But we must all understand that his condition is very serious." He briefed them thoroughly, omitting only the fact that the tumor had been discovered, and ignored, over two and a half years before.

Listening to Johnson's words, Polly felt her mind reel.

John's condition might not be curable! Johnson was not saying so, but that's what he was preparing them for. She glanced at Jack. He was hanging on Johnson's every word. Then, as clearly as if she were reliving it, her son's life flashed before her eyes. She saw him as a cheerful baby, as a youngster playing with his father's two Irish setters. She remembered standing proudly in the doorway as he left for his first day of school; relived endless nights of chicken-pox and measles, rubdowns with cool washcloths, countless glasses of water. She saw him as a teen-ager winning his first race; she heard him cheered across a hundred finish lines. All at once she wanted to rush into the recovery room where her son lay surrounded by strangers and pick him up and cradle him in her arms, to protect him from this nightmare as she had when he was a child. Silently, she prayed for strength, for understanding. No matter how hard this

59

was for her, or her family, or for Mary Ann, it would be horrible for John. She could go to pieces now and become a part of his burden, or she could marshal her resources and do all in her power to help him. She would try.

Johnson had stopped talking.

"Doctor," Polly asked. "When may we see our son?"

Johnson looked at her. He had been right. There was strength there. He looked at his watch. "He should be in his room now. You can go in anytime."

Jack and Polly stood on opposite sides of the bed. The guard rails were still in place. John lay on his back with his head slightly propped by a thin pillow. He looked at his parents. Their faces revealed the anguish they were fighting to conceal.

"You talked with Doctor Johnson?" John asked.

"Yes," Polly replied.

He turned to his father. Suddenly, Jack reached through the railing and grasped his son's hand. "John, I'd do anything, give all I have, to be able to take your place."

John shook his head firmly. "Dad . . . I know." Jack and Polly stayed until John fell asleep.

He sensed someone standing beside his bed. He opened his eyes. Slowly they focused on a familiar figure. "Hey, man," he said, rubbing the drowsiness from his face, "do I ever owe you an apology."

John Haaland shook his head. "You don't owe me anything." He pulled a chair close to the bed. "What's the score, John?"

Baker pushed himself up against the pillows. "It's the big one," he replied matter-of-factly. He went into the diagnosis, the malignant tumor, the extensive surgery to come, what he'd learned from the books at UNM Medical School.

He talked rapidly, incessantly, using the opportunity to discuss things he couldn't with his family. "It's going to tear my folks up," he said, "especially Dad." He paused. "You know, he's always gone to bed at ten-thirty—right after the news. But yesterday morning, at two o'clock, I heard him in the living room and went out. He was just sitting in his chair, staring at nothing. He hadn't even been to bed. I sat down and tried to talk to him, but we couldn't find words. God, it was awful. It's never been easy for him to show his feelings. And now . . . this. It's pure hell for him."

He looked at Haaland resignedly. Haaland was silent, staring at his hands knotted in his lap. Then he looked up. "Say, is there a place around here where a guy can get a cup of coffee?"

John nodded toward the door. "Down the hall. But come right back. Hear?"

"You bet."

Haaland walked down the hall until he was sure he was out of John's sight and sound. Then, he leaned against the wall and began to cry. He had been there several minutes when he heard someone come up behind him. He tried to get control of himself.

"John?"

He turned to see Polly looking at him with compassion.

"You've been in to see John?" she asked.

Haaland nodded. "It's a lousy stinking trick, Mrs. Baker." He shook his head in angry frustration. "What are we going to do?"

John Haaland was like another son to her. For fifteen years the Baker household had been his second home, just as the Haaland household had been John Baker's. And now, more than ever, her son was going to need this special friendship.

61

"John," Polly replied in a steady voice, "we're going to do whatever's necessary to help John face the future. Come what may." She put her hand on his arm. "Starting right now."

He looked at her. If she, of all people, could bear up, so could he. He pulled out a handkerchief and wiped his face. "Wait a second," he said. "I can't go back in there without a cup of coffee in my hand."

John's recuperation from the operation was swift. Wednesday morning, forty-eight hours after surgery, he was home with instructions from Johnson to rest, eat well and build his strength for the big operation to come.

Like Robert, Jill, was also married now and lived out of town. Both were still unaware of John's illness. That evening he decided it was time to make the promised calls. Staff Sergeant Robert Baker was stationed at the Air Force Academy in Colorado Springs. He and his wife Margaret, also from Albuquerque, lived off base. He was delighted to hear his big brother's voice. Though they wrote often, phone calls were rare.

They chatted a few minutes aimlessly. Then, at the first lull, John said, "Bob, I really called to tell you . . . I just had an operation."

"What!?"

"I've got a small cancer. But I don't want you to worry," he added hastily. "It's not the bad kind."

But Robert was immediately concerned. Something in John's voice was unconvincing. "Let me talk to Dad, John," Robert said.

John didn't argue. He called his father to the phone and left the room.

Five minutes later Robert hung up and walked into his living room in a daze. Margaret rushed to his side. "Robert! What's wrong?"

"I've just learned," he said quietly, "that I might lose a guy who means everything in the world to me."

Disturbed by his bungled call to Robert, John asked his parents to call Jill.

"And Mary Ann?" Polly asked.

John shook his head. "No." He didn't elaborate.

The days passed slowly. Restless, full of vigor despite his condition, John took long walks through the parks and golf courses where he used to run. Other days he drove alone to Big U Hill, to sit alone for hours on his beloved mesa. Haaland had left for summer camp with the Army Reserves. To John it was just as well. Though he didn't go out of his way to avoid his friends, neither did he seek them out. To Jack's and Polly's alarm, their once-gregarious, crowd-pleasing son was becoming a loner.

The date for the second operation was set: Tuesday, June seventeenth.

Robert asked for leave, and he and Margaret came home. Jill arrived the next day, alone. For the first time in two years the family was together . The days were devoted to John's favorite foods, favorite haunts, best friends. Touched by his family's efforts, John tried hard to enjoy himself. Slowly, he seemed to emerge from his shell, shoving realities aside. Friends and family alike were encouraged. Except for Polly. With a mother's insight she was not deceived. Though she kept it to herself, she recognized her son's smile for what it was—a mask to hide his anguish.

On Saturday, the fourteenth, Robert announced a surprise. "They're all old friends of yours, John. Buddy and Vicki, Pat, Larry and their dates, Joe and Barbara. And me and Margaret. We'll go to Corrales. Really make a night of it. Just like old times. What do you say?"

They were John's Lobo teammates, or chums from his youth, and their wives and girlfriends. Jill had decided to stay home with her parents.

"Sure, Bob," John agreed. It would help pass the interminable weekend before surgery. "Sounds great."

The rambling, adobe Territorial House nestled near a grove of cottonwood trees on the west bank of the Rio Grande, took pride in its authentic Old West past. Corrales, according to legend, was named in the eighteenth century by conquistadors who pastured their horses there during the Spanish settlement. The Territorial House, built in 1801 on land farmed by Pueblo Indians six centuries before, had been a home, a fortress against marauding Apaches, and a wayside inn. In 1955 the old house was converted to a supper club where customers in jeans could whoop it up to the music of a cowboy band. During his college years it had been one of John's favorite nightspots.

The party glowed. In an outward show of high spirits, John joked with his friends, danced with their wives or dates and joined in endless rounds of chug-a-lug.

Shortly after midnight John stepped outside for air. He strolled deep into the cottonwood grove and leaned back against the trunk of one of the large trees. Across the river, high on the East Mesa, Big U Hill stood bathed in moonlight. Behind the hill, towering above all, was Sandia Crest, the majestic two-mile-high Rocky Mountain peak dominating Albuquerque's eastern skyline. John fixed his eyes on the crest.

In the distance he could hear the band playing. From the club came the sounds of people dancing, laughing, loving. The sounds of life. The sounds of people who could still hope, still dream, still aspire. How remote all that was now. For him there would be no more plans, no more coaching, no more running. And no Olympics. More likely, if his malignancy followed the course he was convinced it would, he and his family faced months of agony.

The towering peak continued to draw his gaze. He had been there many times; had often stood at the edge of the precipice that dropped to the craggy plateau, five thousand feet below. He would go to the mountain tomorrow.

Chapter 5

Sunday, June fifteenth, dawned overcast. The usual crystal-blue sky above Albuquerque was leaden. The temperature was about eighty degrees. On the high mesas whirling dust-devils, whipped by a steady wind, filled the air. It was a day to stay inside.

Polly was disappointed in the weather. She had risen early to begin a special meal for that evening. In two weeks John would be twenty-five. But with all the family home at one time they were going to celebrate early—before the operation. She had hoped this Sunday would be a bright day for John.

From the hallway came the sound of a bedroom door opening. In a few minutes the family would be ready for breakfast. She had already done all she could do this early in the day in preparation for the birthday dinner. She lifted the lid of a simmering pot for one final check before the breakfast rush. Just then she felt an arm slide around her shoulder. Startled, she turned to find John looking down at her. Behind a forced smile, his face was taut.

"Mom, I'm going for a drive . . . by myself."

Involuntarily, Polly shuddered. There was something in his voice. Or his eyes. Whatever, at that moment she felt something sinister between her and her son. For seconds she debated whether to call Jack or Robert. Something restrained her. She forced a smile of her own. "Well, even if it's not your real birthday it is *your* day, to do what you want." She put her hand on his face. "Just . . . take care."

He leaned down and kissed her lightly on the cheek. Without another word he left the house.

Breakfast came and went. Then lunch. The afternoon crept by.

Late in the day, for the second time in a half-hour, Jack went out into the front yard and looked up and down the street. He came back inside damp from the drizzling rain. "Polly," he asked again. "Are you absolutely certain he didn't say where he was going?"

"I'm certain." She shook her head. "Jack, look at you. You're going to make yourself sick."

Robert rose from the couch. "I've had enough. I'm going to look for him."

"Where?" Polly asked.

"I don't know where. The Sidewinder, Corrales, anywhere. It's better than sitting around here stewing. I'll call home every so often, just to check."

Jack hurried to the closet and took out a jacket. "Wait a minute, Robert. I'll go with you."

68

All of a sudden the front door flew open and John's voice boomed through the house: "What's holding up this party? Let's eat!" He stepped into the vestibule and started brushing the rain from his hair. "Hey, Dad . . . Bob, you going somewhere?"

They stared at him dumbfounded. Jack slipped the jacket on sheepishly. "No . . . just a little chilly."

"Good. I want to talk to both of you."

Polly felt her knees go weak. As casually as possible she sank into a chair. Across the room her men were talking cheerfully. But that wasn't all. John was talking to his father and brother about Aspen. He was making plans for his future! Polly's eyes misted. This was not the same despondent son who had kissed her goodbye that morning. For some glorious reason the *real* John Baker had come home.

It was after midnight. The birthday dinner had been a success. But now everyone had gone to bed.

John kicked off his covers. Keyed up, he couldn't sleep. Quietly, he slipped on his robe and went to the kitchen. He turned on the faucet and began to fill the tea kettle. Then he heard someone behind him. He turned. "Why . . . hi! Little sister," he said softly. "Want some tea?"

"I'll make it," Jill replied. She took the kettle from him, finished filling it and put it on the stove. "I thought it might be you out here *trying* to be quiet."

He chuckled. He sat down at the kitchen table and watched her fondly. They had always been close. Trim, darkly beautiful, she was a younger image of their mother. Proudly he recalled how protective he had been of her when she first started turning the boys' heads. Often when

69

he returned from a date before her, he'd wait up for her so they could talk long into the night. They had shared tea on those occasions, too. And confidences. And they had kept each other's secrets.

"Jill."

"Yes, John?" She brought two cups of tea to the table and sat across from him.

He stirred his tea. "I want to tell you something. About today. It's not all pretty. But it's something I want you to know."

In candid detail he told her what he had done that day.

After kissing his mother goodbye that morning he had driven to Interstate 40 leading east out of town. Once outside the city he had pressed the accelerator to the floor. A drizzle had begun. Ignoring the slickened highway, he watched the speedometer climb: seventy–seventy-five–eighty. Seven miles from town he turned north onto Route 10 to Cibola National Forest. Defiantly he whipped the little Triumph along the narrow serpentine road to Sandia Crest.

Just below the summit he came to a long horsehoe turn. At the top bend of the curve he turned onto a rutted dirt road reserved for maintenance vehicles. After a short drive through the tall ponderosas he braked to a stop and left the engine running. Ten feet ahead of him was the barrierless edge of the precipice.

Far below, in the panoramic view of the Rio Grande Valley, were the settings of his life. Despite the overcast he could easily make out Manzano High, where he had begun his running career. Further west was University Stadium, where he had surprised spectators and opponents and won acclaim as the finest miler in New Mexico. To the south was Big U Hill, where he had trained for his Olympic dream. Almost directly below was Aspen Elementary School.

The rain became a steady downpour. He thought about the meaninglessness of his life. Everything had come to nothing. What was left would be the suffering. Not just his own. He thought about Mary Ann—their plans for marriage, children. And his family. He could shorten their agony, and his own, in an instant. The answer lay straight ahead. With a silent prayer he shifted into gear, revved the engine, and released the clutch.

The car lurched forward. Suddenly, a vision flashed before his eyes! Directly in the path of the car stood a group of children. Frantically he braked to a stop. The children were staring at him. Some were weeping. He recognized them. The children of Aspen. The children he had taught to do their best, not to give up. What would his suicide be for them? He switched off the ignition and sat there, crying.

He stayed there for hours, pondering his life. Over and over his thoughts returned to the faces of those children staring at him, questioning him.

The rain stopped. He got out of the car and walked to the cliff edge. Again he looked down at Aspen. Somehow his fears had been stilled. For the first time in three weeks, since his first visit to Doctor Johnson, he felt at peace.

"While I was standing there," he said to Jill, "it all became so clear. I knew then that I'd never marry, or have a family of my own. But I realized something else. I already have hundreds of children. And I made up my mind that whatever comes, what time I have left I'm dedicating to them."

71

They looked at each other in silence.

"Jill . . . do you understand?"

She slid her hand across the table and he grasped it tightly. She had never been prouder of him, never felt closer to him than at this moment.

Chapter 6

Tuesday morning, June seventeenth, Doctor Johnson opened John's abdominal cavity. He found what he had suspected. The tumor was solidly entrenched in John's lymph system from his groin to his sternum. Working deftly, Johnson began the painstaking task of removing the cancerous nodes. Then, to remove malignant cells that might have been dislodged during the operation, he flushed the cavity with sterile water. There was nothing more that surgery could do. Four hours from the first incision Johnson sutured the extensive wound.

At one o'clock the doctor entered the small blue lounge just outside surgery where Jack and Polly sat waiting. He pulled a chair up beside them and dropped wearily into it. The intricate operation had exhausted him. He shook his head slowly. "There's no doubt now . . . it's terminal."

The silence was long. After a while, Polly reached over

73

and placed her hand on Johnson's. He looked at her in surprise. *She* was comforting *him*. Though she didn't speak, the gesture moved him.

"Doctor . . ." The strain in Jack's voice reflected his dread of the question he was about to ask. ". . . can you be more specific . . . about how long?"

Johnson weighed the question carefully. "I have some actuarial charts in my office," he said. "They cover patients in John's category. Perhaps if we went over them together it would help you understand the situation better."

The Bakers looked at each other. "Perhaps in a few days," Jack said.

They never mentioned the subject again.

John turned his head toward the window. The sky was fiery red. Sundown. He looked at the small clock on the table beside his bed. The numerals were blurred. He knew he was still sedated. He remembered hearing his parents' voices. How long ago? They must have been in the room when he was wheeled back from recovery. He glanced around the room again. He was alone now. Just then someone stepped through the door. As the figure came up to his bedside, John saw it was Doctor Johnson.

"How do you feel, John?"

"All washed out," John replied, surprised at the effort it took to speak.

"That's quite normal for what you've been through."

Johnson pulled back the blanket and felt gently along the sides of the bandaged wound. All seemed well. From the corner of his eye he noticed John watching him intently. He pulled the blanket back over John's chest.

"John, the malignancy was widespread. I removed as much of the infected tissue as I could."

There was no noticeable change in John's expression. "How long?" he asked.

Johnson was taken aback. No hesitation. Just the simple laconic question.

Johnson hedged. "All cases are different. It will take . . ."

John shook his head emphatically. "Doctor," he said, "two weeks ago, when you told me this operation would be necessary, you promised to be candid. Remember?"

Johnson remembered. It was a discussion he hoped to postpone until John was stronger.

"Please then," John repeated, "how long?"

After a moment Johnson said, "John, if you respond to the treatments we discussed, the chemotherapy and radiation, we hope to give you some time. If you don't respond, it could be you have as little as six months left."

There was still no change in John. "That soon," he said evenly.

"Yes. I'm sorry."

John's jaw set. "Doctor Johnson. I want those six months. More if you can give them to me." He looked at Johnon. "There's something I have to do."

Johnson returned John's stare. Something about this scene disturbed him. He had performed this sad duty many times. What made this one different? He knew, of course. His patient was accepting the grim news that his life was going to end prematurely with a puzzling equanimity.

"John," Johnson replied at last, "I'll give you as much time as it's humanly possible for me to do."

75

John smiled wanly. Extremely tired, he closed his eyes. "Thanks, Doctor," he said. "That's all I can ask."

The long wound, aggravated by the essential intravenous chemotherapy treatments, would be slow to heal. Late Tuesday night John's pain began in earnest. With varying intensity it would remain with him the rest of his life.

For the first crucial seventy-two hours Polly stayed at her son's bedside, catching fitful moments of sleep in her chair. Late the first night she was awakened by a panicked cry from John's bed. "I'm falling!" He began to thrash about wildly. Polly rushed to the bed and grappled with his flailing arms. "John! Wake up! You're dreaming."

Groggy from sedation he opened his eyes, looked at his mother and lay still. "I was at the peak," he said cryptically. She had no idea what he meant.

She felt a sticky warmness on her hand. Looking down she saw a trickle of blood on John's right forearm. Across the bed an I.V. needle dangled loose at the end of a plastic cord. Although his arm had been strapped to a restraining board his thrashing about had ripped the needle from the vein. Polly rang for the nurse.

Together the nurse and Polly strapped John's arm back to the board and reinserted the needle into the bruised vein. The reinsertion was painful. Fearful he might rip out the needle again while sleeping, John fought the sedative lulling him back to much-needed rest. "I don't want to go through that again."

Polly moved her chair next to the bed and put her hands firmly on his strapped arm. "You go to sleep," she said softly. "I promise I won't let you tear the needle out again."

76

Throughout that night, and the next two, Polly held her son's strapped arm. Only then would he sleep.

Friday morning, three days after his surgery, John woke up early. Deep inside him he felt the constant pain. Seeking relief, he rolled to one side. His eyes fell on his mother. Awkwardly curled in her chair next to his bed she was sleeping a sleep of exhaustion. Her clothes were rumpled. Deep lines marred her face. He gazed at her for several minutes. Then, softly, he called, "Mom."

She didn't respond.

He was about to call her again. Then he recalled an incident from his childhood.

It happened when he was twelve. He was playing with some neighborhood kids on the mesa behind his home and accidentally tripped a girl his same age. The girl was known as a tattletale, and once on her feet she bolted into the Baker house. Polly, who knew the girl's cry-baby reputation, had seen the accident from the bathroom window.

Not bothering to knock, the girl pushed open the patio door and barged into the living room. "Hey, you!" she called out loudly.

Annoyed by the girl's lack of manners, Polly remained in the bathroom and didn't answer.

The girl called out again: "Hey, lady!"

A little better, Polly thought. Still, she didn't respond.

Not to be deterred, the headstrong girl marched through the hallway right up to the closed bathroom door and shouted angrily at the top of her voice: "HEY! SOMEBODY'S MOTHER!"

The incident became a Baker family joke.

Now, gazing fondly at his mother, John propped himself

77

on one elbow and said, "Hey . . . somebody's mother!"

Polly awoke with a start.

"Crank this bed up!" John demanded. "And order me a big breakfast." The "big breakfast" was soft and bland. But with a happy heart Polly watched her son eat his first meal since the operation.

"Mom," John said between bites, "I couldn't have made these past three days without you. But it's time for you to go home and get some rest."

Polly demurred. "There's time enough for that when you're on your feet."

"Mom . . . look at yourself. I bet I could beat you in a footrace down the hall right now. Besides . . ." He lowered his voice conspiratorially. ". . . you can trust me to my panhandlers."

"Panhandlers?"

"Sh-h-h-h." John put a finger to his lips. "That's what I call the nurses."

Polly laughed. Out of relief as much as in reaction to his joke. He did seem much better. Maybe her around-the-clock vigil was no longer necessary. At last she gathered her things, kissed her son's cheek, and left.

John waited until he was certain she was off the ward. Then, grimacing in pain, he rang for the nurse and had her lower the bed quickly. For a horrible moment he thought he might retch. He held his sutured abdomen tightly with both hands. Slowly, the nausea passed. But the fire in his stomach remained. Perspiring heavily he lay back on his pillow and breathed deeply. The sham had tired him greatly, but it had been necessary. He didn't want his mother to have to spend another night in that chair.

The pain continued to tear at his insides. He looked at his

watch. One o'clock. Two hours until his next pain pill. *Should he ring for it early?* The thought annoyed him. He hadn't submitted to having his insides whittled out just so he could spend the remainder of his days on drugs. Then he remembered that in his races every time he had kicked into his final sprint his leg muscles had felt like they were being ripped from the bone. The pain had been unbearable then too. How had he coped? Racing numbers filled his mind. Concentration. He had forced himself to concentrate on the back numbers of the front runners. He had closed his mind to all else. He repeated the word over and over: "Concentration."

On what?

He rang for the nurse and had her raise his bed. At once the fireball in his belly felt like it might explode. The torturous pain demanded his full attention.

"No!" he cried aloud.

Gritting his teeth, he forced his mind onto other things. He recalled stories from his childhood and mentally relived the scenes. He recreated favorite movies, reran cliff-hanging races, recited from memory the record feats of his favorite athletes—George Blanda, Willie Mays, Bob Mathias, Robert Schul. It helped, but not enough.

He thought of Sandia Crest. That bleak rain-darkened day. His headlong rush toward self-destruction. The children who blocked his path. The children of Aspen. How many were there? How many students had he had last year? Four hundred? Five? He began to recite their names, their ages, their descriptions, their likes and dislikes, their strengths and faults, their capabilities, their needs. . . .

"Mr. Baker."

No response.

He felt an arm touch his shoulder. "Mr. Baker. Are you all right?"

He turned to see the ward nurse staring at him with concern.

"You alarmed me for a moment," she said. "You looked as if you were . . . in a trance." She took a small paper cup from her tray and held it out to him. "It's time for your three o'clock pill."

He looked blankly at the cup in the nurse's hand. Had it been two hours? He looked up at the nurse. "Can you just leave it?"

The nurse shook her head. "I'm sorry. It's against the rules."

"Could you hold it for me then? Just in case I have to call for it?'"

The nurse smiled. She put the cup back on the tray. "I'll have it at my desk if you need it."

He never called for it. When pain struck hard he relied on his own antidote—intense concentration. It worked. By ignoring pain he was beginning to control it.

Tuesday, June twenty-fourth, eight days after surgery, John went home. In the mail that morning he received his teaching contract for renewal. He studied the document. The only health question was "Do you have any communicable disease?" Printing a bold "NO!" to the question he signed the contract and remailed it that day.

Despite the month-long ordeal of two operations and sedentary recuperation, John's granite-hard muscle tone remained intact. Eager to stay in shape for Aspen, he began to take long walks. But they didn't satisfy him. Though he increased the distance daily, he remained restless.

One evening after finishing the dinner dishes Polly went to the den. John was sitting on the couch staring into space.

Polly picked up the paper. "There's a new Bergman movie playing in town, John."

No reply.

Polly looked over the paper and shook her head. He didn't even know she had entered the room. He was still staring straight ahead. She followed his gaze and caught her breath. His eyes were locked onto the coat rack in the corner of the den. On the rack hung his track shoes.

Polly spent much of the night worrying that her son might be contemplating running again. It might be disastrous. Somehow, she had to let him know her misgivings.

Next morning after breakfast John carried his tea into the den and noticed his track shoes were gone. He looked around the room and then saw them. Perched side-by-side on the mantel, each shoe contained a bouquet of fresh-cut flowers from the garden. His track shoes had been converted to vases.

It wouldn't work.

John stretched out on his back on top of the examining table. This time Doctor Johnson studied the vein structure in John's arm. With an outsize hypodermic syringe, Johnson withdrew a measured amount of John's blood, mixed it with a proportional amount of Actinomycin "D" and slowly injected the mixture into John's bloodstream. The procedure took about twenty-five minutes.

"We'll do these chemotherapy treatments here at the office just as long as possible," Johnson said. He stood and looked down at his patient. Brow furrowed, John was staring intently at the ceiling. Johnson was getting to know him pretty well. "Lie there until you feel steady," he said. "Then come to the office and we'll talk."

John entered the office and sat down in his usual chair.

Johnson laid his pen on the desk and leaned back. "John, you've got something to get off your chest, haven't you?"

John nodded.

"OK. Let's talk about it."

"Doctor, I've got a girlfriend, my fiancée, Mary Ann Allison . . ." Speaking slowly and thoughtfully he told Johnson in candid detail about Mary Ann, their idyllic days in California, their compatibility, the plans they'd made for their future, their fervent hopes for children. "We were supposed to get married this summer. I haven't called her or answered her letters for over a month now—since I first came to see you in May." He leaned forward and looked at Johnson imploringly. "I've got to tell her something. I . . . please try to understand . . . but, could there be any possibility, any chance at all, that your diagnosis might be wrong?"

Johnson recognized the situation at once. He'd half-expected it before this. John was grasping at the false hope that in his case medical science might have erred. He was pleading for the chance to live, to lead a normal life, to marry and have a family. Johnson didn't relish the professional role the question demanded he play. Even if John had come to him earlier, before the tumor had spread through his system, Johnson would have recommended at least a one-year postponement of marriage. But John's case was far too advanced for even that small hope. There was no doubt he could father children. He wasn't impotent, or sterile. But time to rear a family of his own—no.

Unwilling to prolong self-delusion, Johnson shook his head. "John," he said compassionately, "there's been no mistake. We can't be exactly certain when your time will come. But all tests indicate that it *will* come, far too soon for you to think of a family. As your doctor I must advise you that marriage for you would be highly impractical." He paused a moment. "Do you understand?"

With a deep sigh John sat back in his chair. After a moment he said quietly, "I just don't want anyone clinging to me out of pity."

It was growing dark. Across the UNM campus, lights began to flicker on. Just past the main library John pulled his Triumph into a parking space by the curb. A short walk across the mall he entered Coronado Hall, a student dormitory. In the foyer was a pay phone. He slumped onto the seat beside the phone. He was exhausted. For hours, since leaving Doctor Johnson's office, he had driven around town, trying to bolster himself for this call.

Across the foyer a group of students were having a boisterous bull session. John listened to them a moment. Then, unwilling to procrastinate further, he dialed the operator, transferred the charge to his home phone and asked for Mary Ann's number in California.

Bewildered after a month of no contact Mary Ann responded testily. "Well, John Baker, I'm glad to hear you haven't dropped dead."

John cringed. Then, forcing an even tone, he said, "I've been pretty busy, training and all."

Just then a wave of shouting and laughter rose from the nearby group of merrymaking students.

"It sure doesn't sound like you're training too hard right now," Mary Ann said.

Taking advantage of the unexpected revelry, John said, "I have to play sometimes. Look, Mary Ann . . . I know this is going to be a low blow, but, well, I've been doing a lot of thinking about things. You know, with my Olympic plans and all. And I'm just not sure anymore . . . about a steady relationship, I mean."

There was a long silence. "Steady relationship," Mary Ann said. "John, what are you trying to tell me?"

"I didn't think I'd have to spell it out," John replied.

"John, are you talking about . . . our marriage?"

"Yes." The word almost stuck in his throat.

"John! We've made plans . . . we . . ." Her voice faded for several seconds, then she said, "John, what's wrong?"

"Nothing's wrong," John insisted. "Except that maybe we rushed things. I know it's my fault. And I'm sorry. Really. But, I'm just—not ready . . . that's all."

"John, are you trying to say you don't love me anymore?"

He didn't replay.

"John . . ." she was crying now. ". . . I don't understand."

He knew he couldn't dissemble much longer. "Mary Ann," he said, speaking fast, "there's nothing to understand. It's a mistake. I've just got too many other priorities. And marriage isn't one of them. I'm sorry."

"Other priorities? First you forget to write to me for over a month, and now you tell me you have 'other priorities' . . . As far as I'm concerned, John Baker, you've just moved off *my* priority list for good." She slammed down the receiver.

"Goodbye, Mary Ann," John said quietly to the silent receiver. Then he hung up the phone.

He sat there a moment in silence. Then he walked back across the darkened campus to his car. He slid behind the wheel and fished the keys from his pocket. But his hand was trembling so hard he couldn't insert the key into the ignition. Engulfed by anguish and guilt over the necessary lie, he began to sob. "Why . . . oh, God . . . WHY-Y-Y?" he cried. Unable to control his emotions, he slammed his fist against the steering column so hard one of his knuckles split open. He welcomed the pain.

Following this call, Mary Ann, out of her own pain, made no effort to contact John again, or his family, until the following year, when it was too late.

Polly sipped her morning coffee deep in thought. She glanced at the kitchen clock. Eight o'clock. John had left hours ago. He'd come home late last night and bleakly told her and Jack about his call to Mary Ann. He said he knew he had hurt her so deeply he did not expect ever to hear from her again. He'd sworn them to secrecy, as he later would Robert and Jill. Then, this morning, Polly had heard him rise early and leave without waiting for breakfast.

She finished her coffee and went to the den to tidy the room a bit before she left for work. She began to dust the mantel. Something was amiss. Then, her heart sank. John's track shoes were gone.

The sun was just appearing above Sandia Crest when John parked at the base of Big U Hill. Quickly, he stripped to his track suit beneath his outer clothing and walked to the starting cairn of his measured mile. After several deep breaths he crouched low, clicked his stopwatch to a start and pushed off in his beginning pace. At the finish line he clicked the watch to a stop and dropped to the ground in pain and exhaustion. Gasping for breath he opened his hand and looked at the watch. Almost six minutes! He lay back forlornly. It was over. His previously abundant core of reserve energy—the essential element of champions—was gone.

After several minutes he brought his breathing under control. He walked back to his car and slipped on his clothes. With a lingering glance he scanned his beloved mesa and left. He never returned.

That day, on the lonely mesa where years before it had been born, an old dream died.

It was time for the new dream to begin.

Chapter 7

Veta Mercer listened in stunned silence. It was almost beyond belief. A young, vital man like John Baker in the grip of terminal cancer? Yet, that's exactly what he was saying as he sat across the desk in her office the opening morning of the 1969–70 school year.

"The truth is," John was saying evenly, "I don't know how much time I have left. It could be no longer than Christmas. That's why I want to get it all out in the open with you now, before I get involved in the job. I do want to keep coaching. Very much so. But, under the circumstances, is that fair to you . . . and the children?"

How cruel! Mrs. Mercer thought. Once in every hundred teachers one like John comes along. One with the uncommon empathy to home in on a child's needs, to motivate seemingly hopeless cases. And now this. Mrs. Mercer rose and stepped around her desk. John stood too. She took his hand. "John, I'm proud to have you on the Aspen staff. And *you* will be the judge of how long you can stay."

Knowing that the odds were against his living through the school year, John returned to Aspen and immersed himself in his job with renewed zeal.

Friday afternoon, the end of the first week of school, he dismissed his last class ten minutes early and hurried toward the parking lot. There was just enough time to make it to Doctor Johnson's office for a scheduled chemotherapy treatment. Just inside the parking lot John saw a boy slumped dejectedly against the door of the Triumph. The boy's hands were thrust into his pockets and he was staring vacantly at the ground.

"Hey, Anthony," John said as he got closer and recognized the boy. "Why so glum?"

At the sound of John's voice, twelve-year-old Anthony Straquadine looked up. His face remained solemn. "Coach . . . I've gotta talk to you."

John glanced at his watch. "Well, I'm sorry, old buddy. But right now I just don't have the time. Maybe tomorrow . . ."

Anthony's face clouded over and his eyes returned to the ground.

Glancing at his watch again, John shrugged. He threw the books he was carrying into his car and put a hand on Anthony's shoulder. "Come on," he said. "Let's take a walk and talk."

They crossed the campus to a remote corner of the playground and sat side-by-side in two hanging swings. "I'm not going out for track this year, Coach," Anthony said at last. His voice echoed his hurt.

"Hey, Anthony!" John said with surprise. "That's your favorite sport, isn't it?"

Anthony nodded. "It's this dumb breathing problem I've got. It got worse over the summer. My doctor says it's chronic bronchitis. He's afraid I'll overdo if I go back to running. He says maybe in a couple years. But not now."

John watched the boy's face. He'd seen that look of dejection before in the faces of other children who, for one reason or another, couldn't participate. He knew that being left out could create a negative self-image in the child. *But how do you involve a child in sports who can't run*, he wondered, *or can't throw, or perhaps can't even walk?*

After a while John rose from his swing. It was much too late for his appointment with Johnson. "Come on, Anthony," he said, "I'll give you a ride home."

They drove the ten blocks to the Straquadine home in silence. Parked at the curb, John looked at the unhappy boy beside him. "Anthony," he said, "I don't want you to worry about this anymore. When you come to school Monday I promise you you're going to be a part of the track team."

At the first playground session Monday morning John called for a huddle of all track runners. They mobbed noisily around him. "All right guys, pipe down. I've got an important announcement." He looked over the sea of bobbing heads. "Anthony," he said. "Come up here."

Anthony stepped up beside Coach Baker. "From now on," John said, putting his hand on the boy's shoulder, "Anthony here is going to be my *Student Assistant Track Coach.*" He emphasized the title in official tones. "He won't be doing any running with you for a while. But you

89

all know that he knows the ropes. And he's going to be speaking for me. So listen to him, hear?''

At John's side, Anthony beamed.

John handed the boy a clipboard and pencil. "May as well get started. You coach track this period. I've got to work on some basketball plays with the girls.''

John walked across the campus to an outdoor court where two girls' teams were playing basketball. Joining the play, he frequently looked down to the field below the playground. There, with authoritative aplomb, Anthony put the track groups through their paces. *It was going to work*, John thought. This might be the answer to the full participation he wanted to achieve. But Anthony had been involved in sports. Would a similar tactic work with a student who had never participated in athletics? John decided to find out.

The next morning he walked around the cafeteria building to an alleyway separating the school from the parking lot. At the far end of the alley a young boy stood listlessly bouncing a tennis ball off the school wall. John had been noticing the boy during the first week of school. A fourth-grader, he had enrolled at Aspen that year. From the first day he had made no effort to mix with the other children. Each day when the outside activities bell rang he would retreat to his lonely post in the alleyway. Watching closely one day, John saw that the boy always handled the ever-present tennis ball with his right hand. On closer scrutiny John noticed that the boy's left arm was smaller and shorter than his right.

As John approached, the boy stopped his solitary play. He looked up at John apprehensively. John smiled. "Bill, I need some help. I've been watching you and I think you're just the person I'm looking for.''

90

Embarrassed to have been singled out, Bill fidgeted. "Naw, I don't think so, Coach. I'm no good at sports and stuff." He fixed his eyes on the tennis ball.

"This is different, Bill. Something special." Not giving the boy a chance to back off, John pointed toward the playground where a ballgame was in progress. "See all that stuff out there—bats, gloves, softballs, basketballs and all. Everyday I have to keep track of all that—check it out, check it in." He frowned and shook his head wearily. "It's getting to be too much. I've got to find somebody reliable to take charge of it." He looked back at Bill. "I think you're the person."

Bill looked closely at John. Then, haltingly, he said, "Well . . . I don't know . . . if you think I can."

"I know you can. I wouldn't ask if I had any doubt. But it's a big responsibility. There's a lot of school money tied up in all that equipment. Tell you what. You stick around after classes this afternoon and we'll go over your duties. Can you do that?"

"Yeah . . . sure!"

That afternoon Bill Witherspoon became Coach Baker's "Chief Equipment Watcher."

From that beginning there came into being at Aspen Elementary School a most unlikely children's sports program. With the support of Veta Mercer and his fellow teachers John eliminated from his playing fields the stigma of non-participation. No matter what handicap a child had, there was an esteem-building role for each. Children who had previously stood idle on the sidelines eagerly joined "Coach Baker's Aspen Student Staff," in such rewarding jobs as "Coach's Timekeeper," "Foul Line Supervisor," "Handicap Recorder," "Rollcall Coordinator," and others. New jobs were created to fit each child's particular capability. As a position was established it was posted, with the incumbent's name, on the official Aspen Sports Bulletin Board which John kept on display in the cafeteria. At each posting he ceremoniously awarded the jobholder an official Aspen Jersey. As he slipped the jersey over the child's head the students responded with applause and cheers for the newest member of Coach Baker's "staff."

Soon, around Albuquerque's Northeast Heights School District, children who had never before participated in sports began to tell their parents about a "real neat coach" at Aspen who "depends on me."

Despite his constant battle with pain, John still felt strong. Each day he put on his track shoes and ran with his children. But he realized he needed help if he was to complete his plans for Aspen while he was still physically able. With no funds in the budget for an assistant coach he decided on a novel approach.

The older children he had coached the year before had moved on to Hoover Junior High, right next door to Aspen. One was fourteen-year-old Chuck Lander. Impressed with Chuck's patient manner with the younger children, John had made him a student coaching aide the previous year. Now, once again, he sought Chuck's assistance. If he could work out the details with the Hoover officials, John asked Chuck, would he be willing to help part-time at Aspen. Chuck would be glad to. And his teachers agreed. So Chuck spent his free periods and phys-ed periods at Aspen helping Coach Baker.

Without mentioning his illness, John stressed to Chuck the urgency of full participation for all Aspen students as soon as possible. "One of my biggest problems," John said one day, "is overcoming the inferiority hang-ups some of these kids have. And I sure don't know all the answers. Any suggestions you have in that department will be welcome."

Without hesitation Chuck replied, "Why don't you say something nice about the kids to their parents? The only time parents hear from a teacher these days is when the kids do something wrong."

John laughed, but Chuck didn't crack a smile.

"You mean that, don't you?" John asked.

"Every word," Chuck replied.

John wondered if the boy might have a point. The next morning, during his first free period, he went to the Aspen administration office. He spent the hour thumbing through the "pink slip" file. One after another the comments on these progress reports to parents convinced him Chuck had been right. He replaced the files thoughtfully. Certainly, he agreed, frank progress reports to parents were necessary. But had the schools, perhaps unwittingly, slipped into a pattern of concentrating on the negative?

That afternoon, to Mr. and Mrs. William Witherspoon, Sr., John wrote his first student progress report. In it he praised their son Bill for his help in the Aspen sports program.

From that point on, one afternoon a week, John stayed late at Aspen to write "upbeat notes" to parents. No matter what record a child had in other classes he always found a positive trait or improvement in the child to praise. Assiduously, he ignored the negative.

One afternoon Chuck was called off the playground to Mrs. Mercer's office. Minutes later he emerged from the building pushing a boy in a wheelchair. The boy's right leg,

93

encumbered by a rigid brace, was supported straight out in front of him by a rig mounted to the front of the chair.

Chuck parked the wheelchair beneath one of the few small trees on the barren Aspen campus and waved for Coach's attention. John left a group of runners and walked over to the tree.

"Coach," Chuck said, "this is Bobby Abeyta. He just enrolled today."

John extended his hand. "Hi, Bobby. Welcome to Aspen."

Bobby smiled and shook hands.

John looked at the braced leg. "Accident?" he asked.

Bobby shook his head. "Bone T.B. They're gonna fix my knee next summer. Then I can use crutches."

Each day one of Bobby's classmates would wheel him to a shady spot beneath the small tree. There the crippled boy would enthusiastically cheer whatever game was in progress near-by.

One afternoon John raised his whistle to start a race. Then he hesitated and looked thoughtfully at the whistle in his hand. While the poised runners stared dumbfounded, he turned and walked over to where Bobby was parked beneath the tree. With a flourish John lifted the red lanyard over his neck and draped it around Bobby's neck. Then, grasping the back of the wheelchair, he pushed the surprised boy to the starting line.

"Runners," John announced loudly, "from now on there's going to be a new race starter around here." Turning to Bobby he commanded, "Blow!"

Bobby delivered an ear-splitting blast, sending the runners off in a cloud of dust.

That afternoon, in a spirited ceremony, Bobby Abeyta was installed as Coach Baker's "Official Whistle Blower."

Veta Mercer studied the report on her desk with concern. She pushed a button on her intercom. "Mrs. Radigan. Would you please have Coach Baker come to my office at his first opportunity."

A short while later, John sat casually in the chair across the desk from Mrs. Mercer. Deeply tanned, muscular, he certainly looked fit, she thought. Only someone who knew him well could detect the hint of weariness in his eyes. She picked up a folder from her desk. "John, how many conferences with parents have you had this week?"

John thought for a moment. "Two Monday . . . and two Tuesday—four in all."

"And yesterday," Mrs. Mercer probed.

John's eyes narrowed in suspicion. "Those were in the evening, Mrs. Mercer. On my own time."

Mrs. Mercer nodded. "I understand, John. But, you did meet twice yesterday evening with parents?"

"Yes."

Mrs. Mercer closed the file folder thoughtfully. How could she make her point tactfully? "John, I hope you understand what I have to say. What you've done—are doing—with the children is a magnificient teaching achievement. I'm sure you want nothing to interfere with that. But every day now we're being bombarded by parents with requests for conferences with you."

"What's wrong with that, Mrs. Mercer?" John asked.

"There would be nothing wrong with it—*under normal circumstances.*" She paused to let her meaning take effect.

95

"To be blunt, John, you must start thinking more of your own well-being. You're too important to this school, to these children, for you to exhaust yourself in endless meetings on top of a full coaching schedule."

After a moment John shook his head. "Mrs. Mercer . . . I understand what you're trying to do. And I appreciate it. But I asked to return to Aspen with my eyes wide open. Meeting with parents is an expected part of any teacher's job. If parents ask to see me I'll do what any teacher should. I'll meet with them."

Mrs. Mercer knew she'd failed. Finally, she smiled. "All right, John. Just take care you don't overdo. Will you do that for me?"

He smiled back. "Yes Ma'am. Please don't worry about me."

She waited until she was certain he had left the outer office, then buzzed her secretary. "Mrs. Radigan, I want all future requests from parents to see Coach Baker referred to me personally."

From that day on, without his knowledge, Veta Mercer approved only those conference requests she considered most pressing for him to handle personally. The rest she referred to other teachers or handled herself. As the only person at Aspen, other than John himself, who knew his condition, she was determined to give him as much time as possible to be where he was most needed—with his children.

As his goal of full participation at Aspen neared success, John thought of a new angle to encourage his children. One afternoon he came home carrying two large shopping bags. Curious, Polly followed him to his room and watched him empty the bags onto his bed. Bolts of ribbon material, posterboards, bunting, a stapler, tape, needles and thread, a pair of scissors and an indelible marking pen.

Polly stared at the jumbled pile. "What in the world?"

"Watch," John said.

He sat down at his desk and picked up some of the blue ribbon material. He snipped off two six-inch streamers and made diagonal cuts off the end of each. Next he cut a silver-dollar-size disk from one of the posterboards. To the disk he stapled some bunting, covered it with more of the ribbon material and fashioned a recognizable rosette. He sewed the two streamers to the rosette and held the trophy ribbon up for his mother's approval. "All I have to do is write in the name and what it's for."

The next day at school John began awarding his home-made ribbons to winners and tryers alike. The children responded with glee. Soon, a "Coach Baker Ribbon" was the most sought-after prize at Aspen.

Veta Mercer was not alone in her alarm at John's obsession with his work. As the weeks passed, Jack and Polly, too, grew uneasy. John was staying later and later at school to meet with parents. Weekends he returned to Aspen to work on playground equipment. To Jack and Polly it was an infringement on the time their son had left for himself.

One evening at dinner Jack announced, "John, your mother and I have a surprise for you." He pulled out a letter from his pocket and handed it across the table.

John unfolded the letter and read it. It was notice of a full membership for him at Paradise Hills Country Club where Jack and Polly were members.

"You've always liked the links there," Jack said eagerly.

Wm. J. Buchanan

"We think it's time we started doing more . . . as a family."

"And they've got that fine pool, and terrific restaurant," Polly added. "Dad and I can leave work early most any day. We could meet you at school, and you could ride out with us. Weekends too. It should be great for us all."

John looked at his parents skeptically. For a long moment he said nothing. Then, in a voice almost alien, he asked, "Dad, did you do this to get me away from Aspen?"

Jack cleared his throat. "Well . . . not exactly . . . we . . ."

Polly intervened. "John, it's not to keep you from your job. But you've been *so* involved lately. We just want you to have a place to get away from students and parents at times. A chance to relax. We both think that would be best."

John dropped the letter to the table. "First, Mrs. Mercer . . . and now you," he said cryptically. "Dad . . . Mom. No one means more to me than you two—you and Bob and Jill. You're the only family I'll ever have. But you've got to *understand*. My life now . . . what's left of it . . . is at Aspen. That's the only chance I have to leave anything in this world. I don't have time for Country Clubs, or a fine pool, or anything else." He shook his head. "All I ask . . . is for you to let me live what life I have left in my own way."

He left the table and went to his room.

Jack and Polly sat in strained silence. After a moment Polly laid her hand on Jack's and smiled encouragingly. She rose and went to John's room. "May I come in?"

"Sure," John replied.

He was sitting at his desk inscribing names on trophy rib-

98

bons. Polly sat down on the bed and picked up one of the ribbons. She read aloud: "Bill Witherspoon . . . Chief Equipment Watcher." She picked up another. "Bobby Abeyta . . . Chief Whistle Blower."

She placed the ribbons back on the desk. "John, you work on these ribbons every night. Then you teach school all day. And lately, it seems, you're spending more and more time in conference with parents. Your father and I . . . well, we want what's best for you. And if all this is really worth it . . . "

He reached over and gripped his mother's hand. "Mom, believe me, *it's worth it.*"

Something in his eyes pleaded for her understanding. She squeezed his hand gently. "Well, then, there'll be no more said about it." She picked up one of the unfinished ribbons. "Do you need some help with these?"

John smiled. "You bet." He handed her a pair of scissors and a bolt of ribbon.

With a thankful heart Polly took the items. Each night from then on, when he worked on the awards, she helped her son manufacture his coveted "Coach Baker Ribbons."

One Friday morning Bill Witherspoon came up to John on the playground. "Coach, can you come to your office. You've gotta see something."

He went with Bill to the office. There, seated beside his desk, were two children, a fourth-grade boy and his sister, a second-grader. They looked up through vague, unfocused eyes.

"I found them behind the cafeteria," Bill said. "They're stoned on pot."

99

John moved a chair close to the children. "Where'd you get that stuff?" he asked.

"From Cowboy," the girl blurted before her brother could shush her.

John looked up at Bill.

"He's in the sixth grade," Bill said. He mentioned another school. "This isn't the first time."

Good God! John thought. *Fourth- and second-grade potheads, and a sixth-grade pusher.* He'd deal with Cowboy later.

"Eddie," John said. "You and your sister are on a bad trip. That stuff'll waste your brains. It'll put you out for days."

"Do you smoke pot, Coach?" Eddie asked. He wasn't being insolent.

"No," John replied.

"Then, how do you know?"

John was taken aback. He had no answer.

He kept Eddie and his sister in his office until school was out that afternoon, then sent them home. He didn't mention the incident to anyone.

That afternoon he called a friend at his office. "Martin," he asked, "are you going out of town this weekend?"

A mining engineer, Martin Baccus spent most of his weekends in the uranium country around Grants, New Mexico. John had used Martin's apartment before.

"Hey, buddy," Martin replied. "Sounds like you got something lined up."

"How'd you ever guess?" John said.

"Well, you're in luck. I'm splitting when the whistle blows. You know where the key is. Just wash the damn dishes and try not to burn the place down."

An hour later, on the UNM campus, John purchased six marijuana joints, then drove to Martin's apartment. He locked the door, pulled the blinds, and lit up. On the first drag he broke into a spasm of coughing. He'd never smoked before in his life. When the coughing abated he took a smaller drag. He soon got the knack of it. But at the end of the first cigarette he felt no change. He lit another. He began to despair of getting a reaction. He decided to check the time. When he looked at his wrist he saw two watches.

He moved to a table where he had laid out a tablet and a pen and began to record his reactions. He kept it up throughout the evening. Some of the entries from the log he kept that day read:

This is really happening; tree is dancing; dizzy; giggling; nonsense talk. Went into living room—music by Temp (sic)—feel music in body—out of sight, dancing, groovy, laughing, falling into walls. Mind ahead of body.

At six o'clock he went out to eat. His log reads:

Frank's Pizza; cherry cream pie; food is weird; everybody straight; can't let them know; seems so obvious but nobody noticed.

Back again at the apartment he continued:

Goes in stages, slap-happy, headache, contemplate, no conception of time. Coming down but still up; mouth dry; ate lots of potato chips; love everybody.

101

His last entry was:

Time went so slow, so much happened in the space of one or two minutes, head moved slowly—felt like brotresauraus (sic)—hard to breathe.

Saturday at noon, he awoke and returned home. He found he could barely function. He tried to cut ribbons, but couldn't. It was late Sunday evening before he was able to concentrate on the simplest task.

Monday morning, at Aspen, John began to teach the effects of marijuana on the mind and body. Though classified as a Physical Education Teacher (Coach), he had no formal classroom. So he assembled his children in the large multipurpose room they used for calisthentics in bad weather. He wrote his name and phone number on the blackboard. "If any of you ever get into trouble with this stuff, and need help," he told the children, "call me anytime, night or day. We'll work it out."

Unknown to the children's parents, or his fellow teachers, for the remainder of his time at Aspen, John responded to many such calls for help.

One afternoon in late September John assembled his fourth-grade girls' basketball teams at one of the paved outdoor courts. One of the girls ran up to him. "Show us some free-throws, Coach."

"Sure," he replied.

He stepped to the rear of the court. Holding the ball close to his chest he thrust his arms sharply upward, propelling the ball in a high arc toward the hoop. Suddenly, wincing in pain, he grabbed his left side just below the armpit. He took a couple of deep breaths, looked around quickly and dropped his arm. He was glad the girls had been watching the ball. He called Chuck Lander from another game. "Chuck, take over here a while. I have something to do in my office."

Nonchalantly, he walked across the playground to the administration building.

Seated at a bench near the court, checking his equipment roster, Bill Witherspoon had witnessed the scene. Curious, he put his clipboard down and followed John to his office. He entered without knocking.

John was sitting in his chair sprawled forward across his desk. His head, resting on his folded arms, rolled slowly from side to side. He was moaning.

Bill shivered at the sight. "Coach," he asked timidly, "are you sick or something?"

John raised his head. His face was ashen. His tear-stained eyes reflected an agony the young boy had never witnessed in a person before.

"Bill . . ." John's voice was strained. " . . . close the door . . . come here." With effort he sat back in his chair. "Do me a favor . . . quickly." He spoke fast, between deep rapid breaths. "Get my clothes . . . out of the locker . . . over there."

For the next ten minutes, confused and scared, Bill helped John dress. When they had finished John looked down at the boy kindly. "Bill . . . you and Chuck get the kids in at the end of the period. OK?"

"Sure, Coach."

"And . . . one more thing. Go to Mrs. Mercer. Tell her

103

I'm not feeling well and have left for the day. But please . . . " He looked at Bill pleadingly. " . . . don't say anything to anyone else. No one at all."

Bill nodded his agreement.

By the time John reached the parking lot the pain in his chest had subsided. Nonetheless, he drove straight to St. Joseph Hospital where he had a radiotherapy appointment for later that afternoon.

He explained the sudden attack to the radiologist. Ushered at once to X-ray he stripped to the waist. Peculiarly, now he felt fine—as if the incident had never occurred.

But examination showed otherwise. The X-ray clearly revealed a newly developed mass on his left rib cage. If it signaled a spread of the malignancy to his lungs, then Doctor Johnson's prognosis of six months left for him to live would be tragically confirmed.

The prognosis was already three months old.

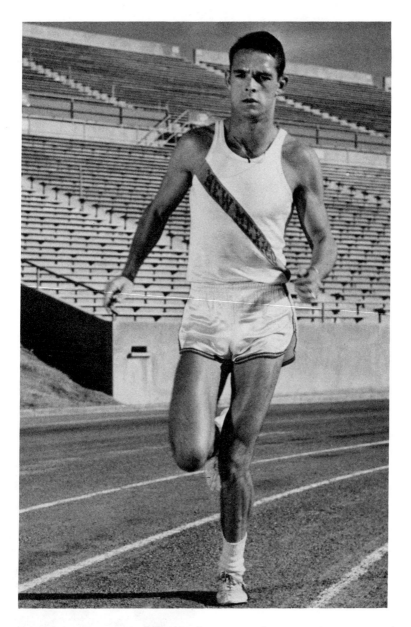

As UNM's star runner, John was by now a prime attraction to sportswriters, touted as "the finest miler ever developed in New Mexico."
Courtesy of University of New Mexico—Richard Meleski.

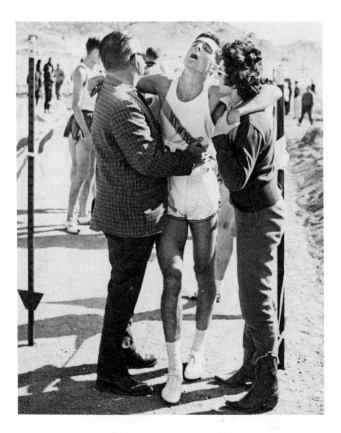

Forcing himself to ignore the fatigue tearing at his muscles, John maintained the furious pace until he crossed the finish line and collapsed in exhaustion. Courtesy of the *Albuquerque Journal*.

Near Big U Hill. Polly Baker said, "You see, I'm the prima donna's mother." Courtesy of Jack Baker.

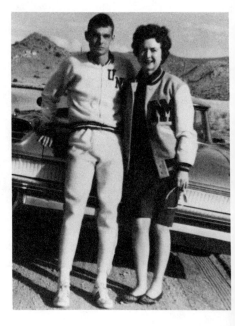

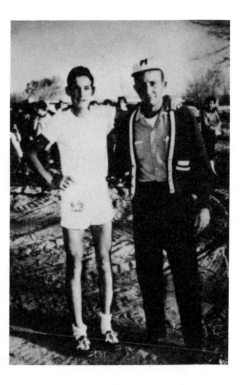

Doubts dispelled, Bill Wolffarth rebuilt his team around Manzano's newest star, John Baker. Courtesy of C. E. Redman.

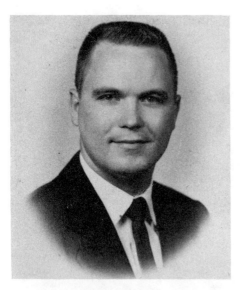

Only a dozen years older than John, Dr. Ed Johnson could all too easily empathize with the younger man.

John made Anthony Straquadine a "Student Assistant Track Coach," knowing that being left out could create a negative self-image in a child." Courtesy of Anthony Straquadine, Sr.

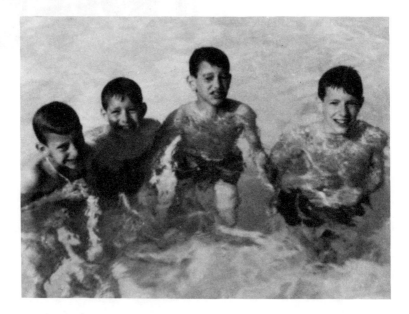

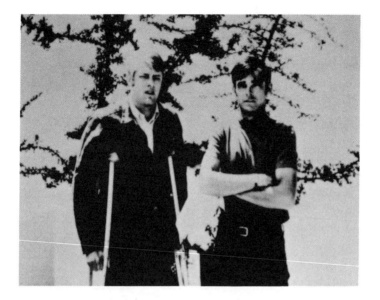

John Haaland on the day he recruited Baker for the Duke City Dashers. Courtesy of Christine Haaland.

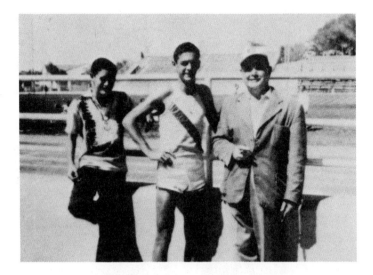

John ended his high school career as the undefeated champion.
With bids from ten universities, he accepted a scholarship from the
University of New Mexico. Courtesy of Polly Baker.

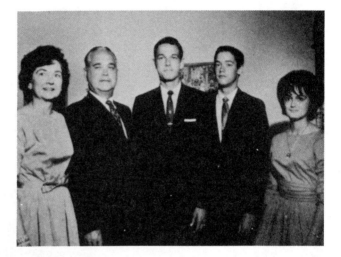

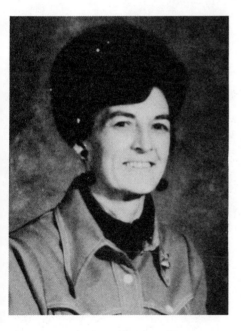

The family had a standing rule: whenever John ran, one or all of them—Polly, Jack Bob, and Jill—would be there to root for him. Courtesy of Smith's Photography.

By the end of that first fall semester, Veta Mercer was convinced that in John Baker she was witnessing a great teacher in the making. Courtesy of Enterprise Studios.

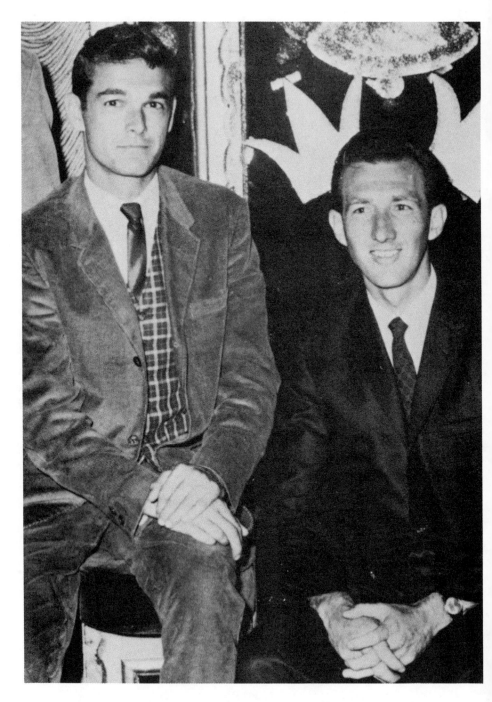

John's final track coach, Robert Schul, said, "I've trained two men who are definitely Olympic caliber. You're one." Courtesy of Athens Athletic Club.

Chapter 8

Chuck Lander woke up. He lay in the darkness adjusting his senses to what had disturbed him. He heard it again. The soft metallic "plink" of a pebble tossed lightly against the pane of his upstairs window. He glanced at his bedside clock. It was 3:45. He knew at once what the clandestine sound meant.

Irritated, he kicked off his covers and went to the window. Sure enough, in the yard below he could see fifteen-year-old Ronald Jones staring up at the window. Ron's motorbike was parked at the side of the house. With a nod Chuck motioned Ron to go through the backyard gate to the rear of the house.

Moving quietly to avoid rousing his parents, Chuck slipped downstairs and opened the backdoor. Ron stepped inside. "OK if I bunk over night, Chuck?" He appeared confident his request would be granted.

In the dim kitchen night-light Chuck sized up his friend. Ron's dress grew more outlandish with each passing day. The legs of his worn jeans were crammed into scuffed, knee-high squaw boots. His bare arms protruded from a sleeveless, imitation-buckskin vest. Beneath the fringed vest, emblazoned on the front of a soiled T-shirt, a clenched fist with the middle finger pointing straight up boldly proclaimed Ron Jones's contempt of the world.

Chuck shook his head. "You dumb freak!" He kept his voice low. "Don't you know there's a curfew in this town for teen-agers?"

Ron shrugged.

Chuck calmed down. This was not the first time he'd let Ron in the backdoor in the small hours of the morning. He motioned toward the stairway. "Another fight at home?"

"What else is new?" Ron replied.

They crept upstairs in silence. Once inside the bedroom Chuck hit the wall switch. In the light he saw that Ron's eyes were inflamed.

"You didn't bring any of that stuff in this house, did you?" Chuck asked sharply.

Ron raised his hands defensively. "Christ, no, Chuck . . . I swear."

Chuck relaxed. "OK. What happened this time?"

Ron sat down on the floor beside the bed and leaned back against the wall. "Same as usual," he said dryly. "I got home about a half-hour ago. Mom was sitting up, waiting for me. At first I thought it was just the time . . . you know . . . three in the morning. But that was only part of it. She started bitching about a call that afternoon from Duncan . . . at school. That shithead's dropping me from class for ditching. How about that?" He looked at Chuck in

106

disgust. "Not because of grades. But because I won't go to his damned class every day."

"Ron . . . there are rules, you know."

Ron made the rude gesture imprinted on his T-shirt. "Up rules!"

The act was unconvincing. The hurt in Ron's voice did not escape Chuck.

"Mom really came unglued," Ron continued. "Called me the same thing you did—a freak,"

Chuck regretted the term.

"She threw an ashtray at me. Almost hit me too. It broke all over the floor." He shook his head. "Jesus. I just took off. Rode around a while. Then came here. Guess that's getting to be a habit, huh?"

Chuck didn't respond. After a moment he went to his closet and took down a sleeping bag. He put it on the floor beside the bed. "Get some sleep, Ron. I've gotta get up in two hours."

Chuck climbed into bed. Maybe it had always been like that between Ron and his mother at home. But in school Ron had always made better grades than anyone. Something had happened. Ron needed help.

"Ron."

No response.

Chuck reached down and shook the sleeping bag. "Ron!"

"Huh . . . what?"

"You going to school today?"

"What . . . naw, man."

"Would you come over to Aspen . . . this afternoon? I want you to meet someone."

Ron sat up. "Man, what the hell are you bull-shitting about? Aspen? I'm in highschool."

"Yeah. But you said you weren't going." Chuck waited a moment. "Come on over. Right after school lets out."

"If it'll make you happy," Ron said. "Now, shut up. OK?"

Doctor Johnson slipped the X-ray film under the retaining clips and switched on the backlight. John could see the outline of the new mass on the film.

"If it resists treatment, John," Johnson said, "it could be critical."

John shook his head. "But there's so much left to do!"

This was the closest Johnson had seen his patient to despair since the second operation. He flipped off the backlight and sat down at his desk. "John, do you want me to brief your parents?"

"No," John said. He didn't elaborate.

The following Monday, while Baker umpired at home plate, two fifth-grade teams played softball. With two outs against the team at bat the next batter hit a slow high fly toward center field. In the outfield eleven-year-old James Lucero signaled for the easy catch—and dropped the ball.

Instantly James's teammates rushed toward him yelling at him. John hurried toward the outfield. As he approached, James slammed his glove to the ground and left the field in a huff. He dropped to the sidelines sulking.

John motioned to Bill Witherspoon. "Umpire for a while, Bill."

John sat down on the grass beside the dejected boy. "Don't you like softball, James?"

James shrugged.

"You like it but you don't play so well, huh?"

James looked up. John smiled. "And sometimes those clowns out there say some pretty tough things."

"Yeah," James agreed.

John nodded. "I know how you feel."

"I bet! My dad's told me about you. You were *always* good."

John denied it. "Not on your life. Of course, I admit that I used to think so. But then one summer I went to California and ran with a man who was really good. He sure found the kinks in my style." He chuckled at the reflection. "But we worked them out. It took time, but I listened to him and I practiced. And together we worked them out."

"So?" James said. "I don't want to play with these guys anymore anyway."

"Oh yes you do," John said. "And I'm getting ready to start a clinic. No stars allowed. Just a session for guys who, well, might be good, but who want to get better. Would you like that?"

"I guess so," James replied.

John smiled. "OK. I'm going to announce it this afternoon." He reached over and mussed James's hair. "And I expect you to show up, old buddy, and practice."

That afternoon John made the promised announcement, and, "Coach Baker's Early-Bird Clinic" was added to his growing roster of innovative programs. Each weekday morning, an hour before school started, John met on the campus with any child who wanted to improve himself in a sport. Chuck volunteered to help. Within a week, a dozen kids had joined James Lucero in taking advantage of the clinic. One was Anthony Straquadine, who, under John's close supervision, started running again to build up his wind. Another was Bill Witherspoon, who discovered that his good right arm provided all the power he needed to become a first-rate softball pitcher.

One morning Chuck showed up late. John regarded him

109

with amusement. "Chuck, you look like something the coyotes dug up."

Chuck yawned. "I didn't get much sleep last night, Coach."

When the bell sounded, Chuck ran over to where Baker was helping Bill Witherspoon retrieve equipment. "Coach, can I talk to you in private?"

"Sure. Grab some of this stuff."

They retreated to John's office. There, Chuck told his coach about Ron Jones.

"We met at Mitchell Elementary, before Aspen was open. Ron was a fun guy to be around then. And he was good in school. But something's happened. He's ditching a lot now. Told me he was about to be suspended. And he's getting spaced out—becoming a real wierdo." Chuck paused. "I thought you could talk to him. You know, like you have some of the guys this year."

John sat leaning back in his chair, feet on his desk, listening. When Chuck finished, John dropped his feet to the floor and said, "Chuck, I've learned that sometimes the best way to help someone is to get them to help you."

Chuck looked puzzled.

"Did Ron ever participate in sports?" John asked.

"Yeah! He used to run. Was pretty good, too."

John nodded. "Good. Maybe we can talk him into helping out here at the clinic. Get him to drop by someday and we'll discuss it."

A sly smile formed on Chuck's face. "He's coming by this afternoon. Why don't we ask him then?"

John laughed. "It looks like I've been set up."

That afternoon Chuck introduced his best friend to his coach. Ron looked disheveled, still wearing the same clothes he'd slept in at Chuck's. Muscular, but lanky, he had a good frame for running. But beneath a shock of dark hair his expression was mocking, chip-on-the-shoulder.

"Chuck tells me you're a runner," John said.

"The best," Ron replied.

John let the boast pass. "He also thinks you might like to help us here at the clinic, before school."

Ron shot an angry glance at Chuck. "Hey, man . . . what is this shit?"

Chuck flushed. "Damn it, Ron, come off it. Coach is asking for your help."

John held up a hand. "It's OK, Chuck. Look, Ron. Chuck tells me you're a good track man. That's fine. If you'd like to come by we can use you. If you don't . . . no sweat."

Ron looked suspiciously from Baker to Chuck and back again. After a moment, with elaborate nonchalance, Ron asked, "When?"

"Any morning an hour before school starts," John replied. Then, deciding to get off on the right relationship from the start, he added, "And Ron, if you do come back on campus, don't wear that T-shirt."

Ron half-opened his mouth to speak, then thought better of it. Raising his hand to his forehead he made a contemptuous salute and strode off toward his parked Honda.

Three mornings later John heard a motorbike enter the campus. He turned to see Ron lean his Honda against the cafeteria wall. As the boy walked toward the field, John noticed that he was wearing the same tattered jeans and vest. But he had on a different shirt.

To Chuck's chagrin Ron made no effort to help out. Each morning the pattern was the same. Soon after the clinic got under way, Ron would ride onto the campus and park his Honda beside the cafeteria. For the remainder of the hour he would stand on the sidelines caustically kibitizing the practice sessions.

John suppressed an urge to ban Ron from Aspen. Something about the boy's braggadocio didn't ring true. Ron Jones was overplaying his act.

One morning as Ron rode away from Aspen, John asked Chuck if he knew anything about the boy's family background.

"Some," Chuck replied. "But my mom knows more. She's known Ron's mom for years."

"Do you think your mother would talk to me about him?"

"Sure. When?"

"Anytime."

"I'll ask her today," Chuck said, "and let you know."

Sunday afternoon, in her home, Katherine Lander, speaking with compassion filled in the gaps in John's skimpy knowledge of Ron Jones. "He was fifteen last June. He has a sister, Kathy, who's nine. Florence—that's Ron's mother—and her husband divorced soon after Kathy was born. Flo never remarried. She moved here to be near relatives."

"She works, then?" John asked.

Mrs. Lander nodded. "She's a legal secretary in an office downtown. It's a good job.

"Ron and Chuck went to grade school together. In the sixth grade Chuck missed a year for medical reasons and Ron got ahead of him. But they remained good friends.

"Somewhere around the eighth grade Ron began to change. He simply started going downhill. You've seen the

112

belligerent way he dresses and acts. Anyway, it soon got to where Chuck was the only one of his friends who would have anything to do with him. It was the same with Ron's schoolwork. He used to be such a good student. But not now."

"You mean the cutting?" John said.

Mrs. Lander nodded. "From what Chuck says, Ron has evidently decided school is a waste of time."

John considered this without comment.

"Mr. Baker . . ." Katherine Lander hesitated. "What I've told you so far is background. And . . . well, Chuck is so excited about what you're trying to do for Ron. I wonder if you'd be interested in my viewpoint . . . in confidence?"

John leaned forward. "I sure would."

For a moment she wondered if she were doing the right thing. Then, she reminded herself of the effect this young man sitting before her had had on her own son. It was worth the risk.

"Since he was six years old Ron hasn't had a father to influence him, or to appreciate and understand his needs as a boy. I've known Flo ever since she moved here and started attending our church. She's truly a fine person and a providing parent. She only recently gave Ron that Honda he rides . . . after one of their arguments. But it's difficult for a mother, alone, to understand a boy who's just moving into adolescence. Especially"—she looked at John tellingly—"when there is a daughter more to her liking. Surely, Ron must resent this. Maybe without realizing why. In my opinion, sometime in the past year or so Ron simply rebelled. It's as if he's made up his mind that if he can't get attention by being a good guy and a good student, then he'll

113

get it by being the opposite. He *is* getting attention. But it's not the kind he really wants. And it's tearing him apart. Ron needs something . . . some accomplishment to take pride in, other than just being a 'tough guy.' ''

It was far more than John had bargained for. After he'd gone to bed that night he mulled over Mrs. Lander's insight. He agreed with her solution. Ron did need a sense of accomplishment to turn him around.

The next morning, unrested after a fitful sleep, John sat on his bed dressing. His eye fell on his trophies. He recalled the thrill of defeating a favored runner. Ron was a runner. What if he happened to defeat a two-time Western Athletic Conference champion? Sense of accomplishment? John hurried through his dressing. He was eager to get to clinic.

A half-hour later, when Ron showed up at Aspen, John asked him to stick around after school started.

At the bell John walked over to where Ron was leaning against a goal support. "Still think you're the best runner around?" John asked jovially.

"I said it—didn't I?" Ron boasted.

John issued the challenge. "Let's find out."

"I don't have any track shoes," Ron said.

"You're wearing tennis shoes. I'll do the same," John replied.

After a moment Ron nodded. "Why not?"

The makeshift dirt track just below the Aspen campus was a 250-yard oval. At the starting line John slowly counted down: "Five . . . four . . . three . . . two . . . one . . . GO!"

The boy was good. Head high, feet planted solidly with each pace, he ran with a near professional stance. On the final turn he kicked into his final sprint. John held his pace.

114

They crossed the finish line almost together, with Ron a half-pace ahead.

John slumped against a dirt bank. He shook his head and smiled. "Whew . . . you *are* good."

Ron smirked. "Like I keep saying, Teach, when you're the best, why sweat it?"

That wasn't pride speaking. It was arrogance. The experiment had backfired. Angrily, John recognized that all he'd done was bolster Ron's inflated ego.

John pushed himself away from the bank. "Come on," he said sharply. "Once more around the track. Just for kicks."

"Are you kidding?" Ron snorted. "Man, you're wiped out."

"You chicken?" John's voice was defiant.

Ron started toward the track. "Let's go," he said icily.

He didn't have a chance. At the signal "GO!" without pacing himself John sprinted all the way. It was Manzano, UNM, and California all over again. Another startled opponent was left behind. John crossed the finish line twenty yards ahead of an astonished Ron Jones.

John collapsed against the dirt bank. This time his exhaustion was real, and painful. In agony he clutched his abdomen with both arms. Each beat of his pounding heart sent spasms of pain through his body. When at last he focused his eyes, Ron was standing in front of him, staring contemptuously.

"So you're a 'superstar,'" Ron said caustically. "Big deal. What's it all prove, anyway?"

The anger John had been suppressing ever since he first met Ron suddenly broke loose. Gritting his teeth against the pain, he pushed himself away from the bank. "What's it all

115

prove? I'll show you what the hell it proves!" He yanked his jersey off over his head and pushed his track shorts down below his navel. The long scar was flushed scarlet from his exertion. Transfixed, Ron stared at the ugly weal that extended from John's upper chest to his pelvis.

"Know what this is?" John asked. "It's where they took out my rotten insides three months ago. And they couldn't get it all. Every step I take, every breath I breathe, it lets me know it's still in there, eating away at my guts. Do you have any idea what I'd give to have your opportunity now? Just to *live*—to make something out of my life?" He shook his head in frustration. "It's crazy. I can't have it, and you're throwing it away." He paused for breath. "What's it all prove? you ask. No need to sweat it, you say. Damn it, kid! Wake up! You can't even compete with a man who's dying of cancer!"

Abruptly John turned and walked off the field. Behind him Ron Jones stared at his departing back.

To John it had been wasted time. Avoiding the details, he told Chuck Ron wouldn't be coming back. "Don't blame yourself," he said. "You did your best. But some people you just can't get through to, no matter how hard you try."

The following Monday morning John pulled into the Aspen parking lot and did a double-take. Ron's Honda was leaning in its usual place alongside the cafeteria wall. It had been seven days since their confrontation.

John parked quickly and ran up the embankment toward the playing field. He raised his hands to shade his eyes and found it difficult to believe what he saw. On the oval track below the campus Ron was helping two of the "early birds" assume a proper starting crouch. While John stood staring, Ron looked up. Their eyes met. After a few seconds, without comment or sign, Ron turned back to his task.

Later that morning, as they walked together toward his parked Honda, Ron agreed to "come by on occasion" and help John at the clinic.

"One condition," John said. "You return to school and attend classes regularly."

Jones shrugged. "I'll try."

"Try?"

"OK, OK!" Ron conceded. "I'll do my best."

"One other thing, Ron. That business last Monday . . . on the track. What I said. Let's keep that just between us. OK?"

For the first time since they'd met, Ron's voice was subdued. "Whatever you say, Coach."

They shook on the deal.

It was not the end of their problems. The agreement they struck that morning would soon be sorely tested. But it was a beginning. And a better one than John thought he'd ever get with Ron Jones.

Chapter 9

Late on Sunday afternoon, October 12, John Haaland came to the end of a stack of documents he was microfilming at Citizen's State Bank where he worked part-time. As he cleared off his desk he glanced up at the wall clock. It was five-thirty. There was plenty of time to get home and spruce up for his date that evening.

At the curbing just inside the bank's parking lot, Haaland's Triumph 650 motorcycle stood shining in the rays of a setting sun. He stooped and looked the bike over carefully. Only a few months before it had been stolen and was found badly damaged. He had put in long hours doing the tedious repair work necessary to restore it to almost new condition. Satisfied with his inspection, Haaland straddled the bike, kicked it to an easy start and merged into the dense weekend traffic heading home.

At the intersection of San Pedro Boulevard and Mountain Road, with the right-of-way in his favor, Haaland continued through the crossing. Suddenly an unexpected movement caught his eye. He looked to the left quickly, and his blood turned to ice-water. A car had run the stop sign and was bearing down on him. In desperation he gunned the accelerator full open. *So this is how I die*, he thought ruefully.

In that instant all went black.

"John."

The voice was hollow, as if it were coming from the bottom of a well.

"John," the voice repeated. "Can you hear me? This is Baker."

Haaland forced his eyes open. Directly above him, surrounded by a strange haze, was the face of his best friend. Haaland struggled to raise his head. "Where . . .?"

Baker placed his hand gently on Haaland's chest. "Lie still. You're at Presbyterian Hospital. You've been in an accident. But they're going to take care of you."

With barely a perceptible nod Haaland lay back on the pillow and closed his eyes. It was the last thing he would remember for four days.

Two hours later Doctor Joseph Hollinger, orthopedist, emerged from the emergency room and joined Haaland's parents and Baker in the same blue lounge where four months before Baker's own parents had anxiously awaited news of him.

"It must have been some impact," Doctor Hollinger remarked.

Mr. Haaland replied, "The police told us it threw him twenty-five feet."

Doctor Hollinger nodded. "John has multiple cuts and

abrasions, and his left shoulder is fractured. But that's not our main concern." Hollinger placed his hands on his own leg between his knee and hip. "In this area John's leg is crushed. It took the full impact between the car and his cycle. The thighbone is severely comminuted—shattered. A few years ago we would have been forced to amputate at once. But now we have an alternative. If we can control the tissue damage we may be able to reinforce the thigh with steel. It will be touch and go. And we'll have to keep John heavily sedated for several days until the operation can be performed. But it's worth the risk to save his leg."

The Haalands agreed to the procedure.

For four days Haaland ranged between feverish delirium and coma. Each afternoon after work Baker came directly to the hospital. He stayed late into the night. Though Haaland was incoherent, Baker talked to him constantly, hopeful that a familiar voice would somehow penetrate Haaland's stupor and bolster his will.

Late Tuesday evening Baker watched the ward nurse check Haaland's vital signs. His bruised head, surrounded by a mass of blonde hair now matted dark with perspiration, lay unmoving on the pillow. He was obviously in a deep sedated sleep.

Baker rose to leave. "If he happens to waken," he said to the nurse, "tell him I'll be here tomorrow morning for the operation."

He realized he was hungry. A short drive from the hospital he turned onto a side street near the University. At the end of the street, in front of a converted antebellum home, a red neon sign proclaimed "Sidewinder Tavern." He parked in the gravel lot beside the building and walked through the tavern to a high-back booth just opposite a

121

small bar. He'd come here often when he was going to the University.

He ordered a pizza and sat back in the cozy security of the booth to relax. At the end of the bar a television set was tuned to a comedy show. He watched the show until his meal arrived.

The pizza was tasty. He ate heartily, surprised at his hunger. Then, he glanced up at the television—and froze. The program had changed to a medical drama. On the screen a harried surgeon was working frantically over the victim of some unknown trauma.

He rose from the booth, walked over to the television and jabbed the "off" button. He stood there a moment looking at the blackened screen. Then he looked around the room anxiously. The other customers were oblivious to the moment.

He returned to the booth and pushed his food away. "Damn!" he said quietly. He was sick of it all! Hospitals, doctors, illness . . . death!

He rose and walked through the wide arched doorway into the candle-lit lounge on the opposite side of the bar from the dining room. He took a table in a secluded corner. His mind was a jumble of questions. Outside of his family he had mentioned his illness to no one except John Haaland, Veta Mercer, and, almost by accident, Ron Jones. Why, now, did he feel a compelling need to cry out to anyone who would listen: "I've got terminal cancer!"? He shook his head. Never a heavy drinker, he ordered a glass of sherry. Then, oblivious to his surrounding, he sat in thought, staring blankly at the amber wine.

A pair of soft hands clasped themselves over his eyes.

Startled, he sat upright and started to pry the hands away.

"No fair!" a female voice behind him cried. "You've got to guess who."

The lyrical voice triggered a lovely image in his mind.

"Dianna!" he said.

The hands dropped away. "Spoilsport," the voice said petulantly.

He turned around. As he had guessed, a small, dark-haired woman stood smiling at him impishly. He jumped up and hugged her. "Where's Ralph?" he asked.

Dianna Briggs sighed. "At the moment he's somewhere between San Diego and Southeast Asia on a destroyer." She shoved her left hand near the candle on the table and a diamond solitaire glittered in the flickering light. "But when he comes home he's going to be all mine."

"Hey! About time," John said enthusiastically. He stepped back and looked the girl up and down. She was dressed in custom-tailored jeans and a matching denim jacket. In proud deference to her Navajo grandmother, her raven hair was pulled straight back, dropping in a single well-brushed fall between her shoulders. John nodded approvingly.

"Are you alone?" he asked.

Dianna nodded toward the doorway. Two other girls stood patiently watching the reunion. "We just finished dinner," Dianna said. "We were on our way out when I spotted you over here all by your lonesome. I made them wait while I came over to say 'hi.'"

John glanced at the waiting girls again. "Dianna . . . are you going anywhere special, you and your friends?"

"No. Not really."

"Would you stay a while, then? For old times' sake. I'll drive you home whenever you say."

Something in his voice disturbed her. She wasn't afraid. She knew him better than that. But he seemed somehow to be appealing to her.

She turned and walked over to her friends. In a moment they nodded and left. She returned to the table and sat down across from him. "How long has it been, Dianna? A year? Two?"

"Over two," she replied. "Since graduation."

"Graduation," he repeated softly. "We had some great times, didn't we?" he said wistfully. "The track meets, the proms, those picnics in the mountains. You and Ralph, me and . . ."

"And *whoever*," she interrupted with a mischievous grin.

John laughed. "Don't exaggerate."

"Who's exaggerating?" Dianna retorted.

"OK, OK. But tell me about yourself. Are you still acting? Surely Hollywood has called by now."

"Oh, no," she replied. "Nothing that glamorous. I still do Little Theater from time to time. Some assistant directing whenever I get the chance. But mostly"—she lifted her ring finger—"just waiting."

John reached across the table and touched the ring. "I'm happy for you, Dianna. I mean that, really."

He grew silent, and his eyes remained fixed on the ring. In the dim light Dianna studied him. He hadn't changed much. A little thinner, perhaps. She had known him—how long? Ten years? At least. Ever since highschool. He'd been a track hero at Manzano, and later at the university. He'd had dozens of girlfriends then. And the guys liked him

124

too. He and Ralph had been buddies. Those had been good years. And in all that time she had never seen John Baker down. But he was down now. A romance gone awry? The end of an affair? She suspected something like that.

"John," she said softly. "Would you like to talk about it?"

She seemed to be inviting his confidence. "Yes, I would," he said. "But not here." He pushed back his chair and reached for her arm. "I'll drive you home. We can talk on the way."

An hour later he pulled his sportscar into the gravel driveway of a large adobe hacienda in the Sandia foothills and shut off the engine. It had been a circuitous drive to Dianna's home. She sat beside him now in silence, staring solemnly at her hands cupped in her lap. After a long while she took a deep breath and let it out slowly. "I never dreamed anything like . . . that," she said. "But I'm glad you told me."

He looked at her fondly. "I am too, Dianna. It's helped. It really has."

"The only thing I don't understand," she said, "is, why me? Surely you must have plenty of girls to talk to."

"No," he said. "I don't date anymore. It's too complicated, trying to ignore reality, or explain it. I can't stand the thought of a relationship based on pity. And I'd always be wondering. But with you it's different." He reached over and lifted her ring finger gently. "You have Ralph. Your commitment has been made. I can talk to you freely, Dianna. Without worrying about getting involved." He looked at her hopefully. "Does that make any sense?"

"I understand," she said softly.

"I can call you again, then?"

125

"Anytime you feel like it, John."

He walked her to the door. As he had in the tavern, he hugged her closely, and this time kissed her lightly on the cheek. "Thanks, Dianna."

She nodded silently.

She stepped inside and leaned back against the door, listening to the sound of his car recede in the night. Tears ran down her face. She went into the unlighted living room, dropped into a chair, and let them come freely.

"Madre de dios," she whispered into the darkness, crossing herself, "help me to do what I can to ease his suffering." She paused a moment, then added fervently, "and help me not to become involved."

Chapter 10

Wednesday morning, three days after John Haaland's accident, Doctor Hollinger repaired his shattered femur with a twelve-inch steel plate anchored to the bone between his hip and knee. He would remain hospitalized for two months, and be convalescing at his parents' home for two more months. But the operation would prove a success.

For the first three weeks of Haaland's crisis, to Doctor Johnson's consternation, Baker discontinued his chemotherapy and radiation. He feared they would leave him too nauseated to help his friend. But with Haaland on the mend, Baker resumed the treatments. The chemotherapy injections were still performed in Johnson's office. For radiation Baker reported to the radiology clinic at St. Joseph Hospital in Albuquerque. There, in a lead-shielded room, he lay naked beneath a sheet on a narrow table while above him a massive cobalt gun directed a precise stream of gamma rays over a wide area of his body. The treatments took thirty minutes, twenty-two minutes longer than those the average cancer patient received.

One afternoon John came home from a treatment at St. Joseph and dropped limply onto the couch in the living room. Polly came out from the kitchen and saw he was lying curled on one side with his eyes closed. As always following radiation treatments, he was sickly pale. His breathing was fast and shallow.

Polly debated mentioning the note she held in her hand. Deciding against it, she shoved the piece of paper into her apron pocket and started back into the kitchen.

"Mom, what's that you had in your hand?"

Polly turned and reluctantly withdrew the note. "You've had several calls from Ron Jones. He sounded upset. He left this number."

John reached out and took the note. He recognized Chuck Lander's number.

Still unsteady on his feet, he went to the kitchen and dialed. Mrs. Lander answered.

"Ron's out back with Chuck right now, Mr. Baker," she said. "I think it's some problem at his school. Anyway, he's been here all afternoon and won't go home until he talks to you. If you'll hold on a second I'll call him."

John had learned that his students were often more open with him if he met them in places familiar to them. He suspected it would be the same with Ron.

"If it's all right with you, Mrs. Lander," he said, "I'd just as soon come over. I can be there in a few minutes."

128

"Certainly it's all right, Mr. Baker. I'll tell the boys you're on your way."

The two boys met him at the garden gate and led him to a wooden bench beneath the huge elms in the Landers' backyard. They pulled lawn chairs close to him. Chuck stared at John, puzzled by his gray pallor.

"Are you OK, Coach?" Chuck asked.

"Just a little under the weather," John replied. "Chuck, I wonder if your mother would fix me a cup of tea, real hot?"

"Sure." Chuck ran toward the house.

John turned to Ron. "OK, Ron. What's up?"

"I'm dropping out of school, Coach. I wanted you to know first, because of our deal."

"Do you mind telling me why?" John asked.

"It's that damned Duncan," he said. His voice was a mixture of pain and defiance. "I can't take his crap anymore."

"Emmett Duncan?" John asked.

"Yeah. That's him. You two are friends, I guess."

"I know him," John said. "What's the gripe?"

"He's the one who kicked me out of his English class last month. Then, after my deal with you, he didn't want to let me back in. I had to almost beg. I told him about working with you and Chuck at the clinic and that I'd promised you I'd go back to school. He finally said OK, but that I'd have to do some make-up work. I expected that. He really poured it on too—a whole semester thesis on American Lit due in four weeks. I knew he was trying to shovel me under. But I did it. I worked hard on it, too. You can ask Chuck. He'll tell you."

129

"I believe you, Ron."

"Well, I turned it in yesterday. Know what Duncan did? He called me in this morning. Said it was one of the best papers he'd ever read. Really greased me up. Then he said that if anyone else had done the paper he'd give them an 'A.' But he wasn't giving me an 'A' because I didn't deserve one. He's giving me a 'C'!" Ron's voice was bitter. "That's unfair as hell, Coach. Sure, I goofed off. But I did his damned make-up work. And if it's an 'A' paper then I think that's what I deserve. But Duncan doesn't. So, I'm not going back." Barely managing to maintain his forced bravado, Ron sat forward on the edge of the chair and tried to read the reaction in John's face.

With a weary sigh John leaned his head against the back of the bench and closed his eyes.

Chuck arrived with a steaming cup of tea. John sipped it slowly, thankful as the scalding liquid soothed the agony deep inside. As last he leaned forward and looked Ron straight in the eye. "Ron, are you telling me the complete truth?"

"I swear, Coach!" Ron blurted. "Just go ask Duncan."

John sat back and nodded. "That's exactly what I intend to do," he said. "Tomorrow. And I don't want you to do anything else about it until you hear from me again. Got that?"

Relieved, Ron agreed.

Emmett Duncan listened as John explained his reason for requesting their meeting. They sat alone in the teachers' lounge at a Northeast Heights school, just after the last afternoon class had been dismissed. A large, portly man, with prematurely gray hair and sallow skin, Duncan appeared older than his twenty-six years.

As John finished talking, Duncan nodded. "Essentially it's as Ron told you," he said. "Except he conveniently omitted telling you my reason, which I explained to him fully."

"I'd like to hear it, Em."

"Simple," Duncan said. "Fairness."

"Fairness to whom, Em?"

"To my other students," Duncan replied. He leaned forward in his chair. John's tone was beginning to annoy him. "Look, John. Ron told me about your deal. I can appreciate your concern. But, frankly, I think you've taken leave of your senses. Ron is bad news. A twenty-four-carat troublemaker. I deal with creeps like him everyday. If you must know, I find him a pain-in-the-ass. OK, so he did some good make-up work. First honest effort he's put out in months. But how could I possibly justify giving an 'A' to a student I suspended from class only four weeks earlier? You answer that."

"You could justify it because he did 'A' work," John replied.

"No way, John. Use your head. Can't you just imagine how that would go over in admint?"

"Admint?" John asked. "What's admint got to do with this?"

Duncan's voice rose. "What's admint got to do with it? Come on, fellow. This is old Em, your beer-drinking buddy from highschool and college, remember? You know the score. We both work for the same system. Who do you think writes those make-or-break efficiency reports that go

131

in our personnel files? You know damn well what admint has to do with this.''

Striving to keep his voice even, John replied. ''Em, I didn't come here to discuss your career. I'm here to talk about a bitter, confused kid who's crying out for help even if he doesn't realize it himself. This grade—one he's earned fair and square—could go a long way in helping him get his priorities back in order.''

Duncan pushed back his chair. ''John, I don't know why you're suddenly compelled to walk in where angels fear to tread. That's your business. But what I do in my class is mine. I'll give Jones the grade *I* think he deserves. And he can accept it, or go suck his thumb. I'm not a father confessor. I'm a teacher.''

After a long moment, John shook his head solemnly. ''No, Em,'' he said icily. ''Whatever you are, you're no teacher.'' No longer trying to disguise his anger, John stood and walked out of the room.

As he drove home his anger turned to introspection. Something Duncan had said stuck in his mind. What was it? '' . . . you're suddenly compelled to walk in where angels fear to tread.'' *Had the cancer*, John wondered, *the certainty of his fate, made him bolder in standing up for his students than he would have been otherwise?* He hoped not. But that was an issue to think through later. The issue now was what to do about Ron Jones.

There was another approach. It would be hard to bring off. But with the help of someone who had been in the school system a long time, and knew the ropes, someone who would be sympathetic, maybe he could get Ron transferred to another highschool. The idea perked him up. He

132

knew just the person to approach. His old coach, Bill Wolf-farth, was still teaching at Manzano. If anyone could help, he could.

After dinner he waited until his mother had finished the dishes, then went to the kitchen to call Wolffarth. He reached for the phone just as it rang. To his surprise Emmett Duncan was on the line. "John," Duncan said brusquely, "I want to talk to you. I'll meet you at the Sidewinder in thirty minutes."

As usual the tavern was crowded. In the lounge, the dance floor was packed with university students dancing to the beat of a hard-rock trio. John picked out Duncan sitting at the end of the bar next to the dining booths. His Scottish Tartan snap-brim cap was on the stool next to him. John walked over, picked up the cap and sat down. "Hi, Em. Here's your hat."

Duncan raised a stein of beer. "Name your poison. I'm buying."

John motioned to the bartender. "Tea, Gus. Real hot. OK?"

"You got a bug or something, John? You didn't look too good this afternoon either."

"Something like that, Em."

Duncan sipped his beer. After a while, without looking up, he said plaintively, "That was a pretty tough blow this afternoon, John. You hit me where I live."

"I'm sorry, Em. But I was calling it like I saw it."

Duncan nodded. "I was going to be Mr. Chips too, you know, once upon a time."

John let it pass.

"Look, John. I've got forty-four kids in my class. That's

133

twice as many as any teacher is capable of handling efficiently. And it's not like in our day. I remember getting the boot from study hall once just for chewing gum. Christ, John . . . I've got kids in class who are mainliners! I don't have time for tea and sympathy, or for being innovative. I just follow the rules the head-shed hands down."

John sipped his tea, waiting for the bottom line.

Duncan drained his beer stein, set it down roughly and turned half around on his stool facing John. "OK," he said abruptly. "Jones gets his damned 'A.' But if there's any repercussion from this, any bitch at all, you're going to the front office with me. You got that?"

John almost choked on a mouthful of tea. He set the cup down, swallowed hard and looked at Duncan in surprise. "Em, that's great! You bet I'll go with you if you get any static."

"And another thing, friend," Duncan continued. "I'm not the only one who's going to crawfish on this. Jones is going to have to come to class regularly. And he's going to have to work. He's proved he's capable, so there's no excuse for him not to keep it up. Furthermore, from now on, when Jones speaks to me, or to any other teacher, he's going to say 'Mister' or 'Miss.' That's part of the bargain."

John felt good. The pain was still there, but he didn't care. He slapped Duncan on the back. "*Mister* Duncan," he said good-naturedly, "you've got yourself a deal. And if Jones ever breaks it, or even bends it a little, I want to hear about it fast."

Duncan smiled wryly. "Oh, you will, John. You will, indeed."

The next morning Ron Jones sat in front of John's desk

134

shaking his head forlornly. "*Mister* Duncan?" he said dejectedly.

"That's right, Ron," John replied. "And you'll say it with a smile." Inwardly amused, John watched Ron's face contort in feigned agony. It was a good show. But the boy was relieved.

It's going to be all right, John thought to himself, happily.

Chapter 11

Veta Mercer picked up the letter from her desk and read it through once more, concentrating on the final paragraph:

> I doubt if any mother who has not personally experienced the bitter helplessness of seeing her child on a self-destructive path could truly appreciate what Mr. Baker has done for Ron. I know of no better example of a man standing tall by stooping to help a child. I intend to tell Mr. Baker this personally, but I wanted you to know about it too.
>
> Sincerely,
> FLORENCE JONES

Mrs. Mercer rose from her chair and stepped out to her secretary's office. She handed the letter to Mrs. Radigan. "Have you read this one, Jeanne?"

Mrs. Radigan nodded. "Yes. It came this morning."

"How many does this make?" Mrs. Mercer asked.

Mrs. Radigan thought a minute. "At least twenty. Maybe more. I've been putting them all in John's box."

"Jeanne . . . has Mrs. Baker ever mentioned any of them to you?"

"Why . . . no, come to think of it, she hasn't."

"Hmmm. All right. Thanks, Jeanne."

Mrs. Mercer went back to her desk and looked over the notations on her calendar. There were still many things to do before the Thanksgiving Vacation started the next day. She picked a file folder from her in-basket and began to check the entries. But her mind wouldn't focus on the task. She closed the folder and sat back in her chair, mulling over the letters about John Baker she had received from parents over the past month. She couldn't recall a similar outpouring of praise for a teacher in her career. The staff at Aspen referred to the avalanche of letters as "Baker's fan mail." Mrs. Mercer thought it was odd that Mrs. Baker, whom she had seen at several school functions, hadn't mentioned them. That was unlike her. Could it be John's parents didn't know about the letters?

Mrs. Mercer again went to the outer office. Mrs. Radigan wasn't at her desk. Standing against the wall by the door was a high cabinet with pigeon-hole receptacles, each marked with a teacher's name. The letter from Florence Jones was in the box marked "BAKER." Mrs. Mercer pulled out the letter and took it to her office. Picking up the phone she dialed John's home number. As she hoped, Polly answered.

"Mrs. Baker, this is Veta Mercer. I have something here I'd like to read to you if you have a moment."

"Certainly, Mrs. Mercer," Polly replied.

Mrs. Mercer read the letter from Florence Jones.

There was a pause on the line. Then, obviously touched, Polly said, "What a marvelous thing for her to do. Would it be possible for me to get that letter? I know Jack would love to see it."

So I was right, Mrs. Mercer thought. "Yes, certainly," she said. "By the way, has John ever mentioned any other letters like this to you?"

"Why no," Polly replied. "Have there been others?"

"Many others. Some addressed to me, others to John directly. Mrs. Radigan has been putting them all in John's correspondence box. I can't imagine why he hasn't mentioned them to you."

There was another pause. "Mrs. Mercer," Polly said, "I think I know why John hasn't mentioned the letters. And I also think I know where they might be. I do thank you for telling me about them." She hung up the phone and remained seated at the kitchen table. She couldn't find out if her guess were right until that evening. But if letters praising her son existed she certainly wanted to find them.

Dinner passed slowly. With forced interest Polly listened to Jack and John comment about their day, but her mind was on something she had to do, casually, so as not to raise suspicion.

When Jack and John had settled in the living room, each with a section of the evening paper, Polly carried the dinner dishes to the kitchen and put them in the sink. Then she grabbed the almost full bottle of dishwashing liquid from the counter top and stashed it under the sink. "Oh, darn!" she wailed, loud enough for her voice to carry.

"What's wrong, hon?" Jack called from the living room.

Polly came out of the kitchen, taking off her apron. "Oh,

139

I'm out of dishwashing soap again," she said disgustedly. "John, would you lend me your car for a few minutes?"

John laid the paper down on the couch and stood up. "I'll go, Mom," he said.

"No," Polly said hastily. "I've got to pick up a few odds and ends. You stay here and read."

"OK." He handed his mother the keys.

She drove the Triumph to the nearest shopping center and pulled up under one of the bright parking-lot lights. She got out, walked to the rear and opened the trunk. As she suspected, the tire well was littered with papers, books and charts. As he had all through college, John was still using his car trunk as a personal filing cabinet.

Quickly, Polly sorted through the jumbled papers. On the bottom of the pile she found a letter addressed to Veta Mercer. Nearby was another, and still others, some to Mrs. Mercer, some to John. In five minutes Polly retrieved twenty-two letters from the littered trunk.

She went into the store, bought a bottle of detergent and had the clerk put it in an oversize sack. Back at the car she put the letters in the sack along with her purchase. Eager to study her find, she drove home hurriedly.

She did the dishes quickly, then excused herself to do some work in her bedroom. She locked the door quietly and emptied the sack of letters onto her bed. Some were written in ink, some were typed, others were scrawled with pencil. The first one she picked up was from the mother of a ten-year-old boy:

My son was a morning monster. Getting him up, fed and out the door was an almost unbearable burden. Now, he can't wait for school to start each day. He's Coach Baker's Chief In-field Raker!

140

Polly opened another letter:

Despite my son's assertions [another mother wrote] I couldn't believe there was a superman at Aspen. One morning I drove over secretly to watch Coach Baker with the children. My son was right.

A prominent community leader, a father, wrote:

When I get discouraged with the moral decline I see all around us today I think of your unselfish devotion to our children; your efforts to build rather than to put down; your efforts to help our children develop self-discipline; to increase their tolerance of the limitations of others; to learn the value of a positive self-regard. Your influence will help my daughters for the rest of their lives. You have my utmost admiration. I salute you.

And from two grandparents:

In other schools our granddaughter suffered terribly from her awkwardness. Then, this wonderful year at Aspen, Coach Baker gave her an "A" for doing her best. God bless this young man who gave a timid child self-respect.

One by one the remaining letters, each in its own fashion, proclaimed the same hearfelt message.

Polly's eyes filled with tears. She picked up all the letters at once and clutched them tight to her breast. For the first time in months her control over her emotions failed her. Still clutching the letters tightly she fell back on the bed and let the bittersweet pride that had welled within her vent itself in silent weeping.

She lay there for a half-hour, dwelling lovingly on the expressive tributes to her son. She knew John had been touched deeply by the letters or he would not have saved them. But to speak of them openly would embarrass him. She decided not to mention them unless he did first.

At last she rose from the bed, went to her closet and took down an empty shoebox. She put the letters in the box and placed it back on the closet shelf. She made a mental note to talk to Jack about them later.

That box would be joined by many others, all bearing similar contents. For in the course of a year over five hundred letters and cards would arrive at Aspen, or the Baker residence, from grateful parents who recognized that in John Baker a remarkable influence for good had touched the lives of their children.

Chapter 12

Polly opened another bag of mulch she had saved from summer grass clippings and spread it generously over the back-yard flower bed. She spaded the mulch in deep to catch and hold the winter moisture. In these hours of working in the garden she could reflect on the course of her life, and the lives of those she loved. Her thoughts this sunny afternoon centered on Thanksgiving Day, now four days past, when the whole family had gathered again. It had been unexpected, because this year Robert and Jill had been scheduled to spend the vacation day with their in-laws. Their change of plans was accepted without question or comment. For it was understood by all that each day Robert and Jill could spend with their brother was precious to them.

From the driveway in front of the house came the screech of tires braking to an abrupt stop. A car door slammed. Moments later the front door of the house did likewise. "Mom!"

"Out here, John."

John came bursting through the patio door. Without a word he rushed over to his mother, threw his arms around her and hugged her so tightly that he lifted her off the ground.

"John! You're squeezing the breath out of me!"

He set her down gently. Then, barely able to contain himself, he held her at arm's length and gazed at her intently. "Mom. The mass is gone!"

"What!?"

"Gone. Vanished." He moved his hand in a small arc over his upper left chest. "There's no indication of it on the X-ray. Absolutely none! Mom, do you know what this means? I might lick this thing after all!"

Polly felt the strength drain from her legs. "John, let's get out of the sun."

They went to the sheltered patio and sat beside each other in the glider. Polly's heart was pounding. She didn't know if she were going to laugh or cry. Her son was euphoric. At last, taking a deep breath, she forced herself to ask as calmly as possible. "John . . . now tell me exactly, what did Doctor Johnson say?"

"Oh, I haven't told him yet. I've just come from Saint Joseph. The X-ray technician showed it to me on the film. Mom, isn't this great?"

A chill shot through Polly. *Oh, dear God, no!* she thought. An X-ray technician! She fought to get a grip on her conflicting emotions. She didn't want to dash her son's first ray of hope in months. But how cruel this could be if it were not true. She reached across the back of the glider and

144

put her hand on John's shoulder. "John, I'm so happy for you. For all of us. But, really, shouldn't you discuss it with Doctor Johnson?"

"I will, Mom. I promise." He jumped to his feet. "But right now I've got to go to the hospital and tell Haaland. I can't wait to see his face when he hears this."

He bent low and kissed his mother on the cheek. "Tell Dad I'll explain it all when I get home. OK?"

"OK," Polly repeated as cheerfully as possible.

She watched him bound around the corner of the house heading for his car. She remained on the glider, her thoughts a mixture of hope and foreboding. After a while she got up and went inside. No more yard work today. She settled on the couch to wait for Jack to come home. "If only it could be true!" she said to herself fervently. Over and over in her mind she repeated the prayerful plea.

The next morning when she stepped out for the paper, she stopped short. John's Triumph was parked three feet from the curb with the back angling out into the street. An empty champagne bottle lay on the front seat. Polly smiled. "Why not?" she said to herself. She returned to the house for John's car keys and parked the Triumph in the driveway.

December came. In a burst of activity John exhumed plans for his future he had ruefully cast aside. First among them was a hasty application to the University of New Mexico for graduate studies in Physical Education. "Mom," he told Polly excitedly, "as soon as I graduate I'm going to establish a clinic for training handicapped children in sports."

Despite his earlier promise, he repeatedly begged off go-

145

ing to see Doctor Johnson about the X-ray. As the days passed Polly grew more alarmed. It was as if her son had convinced himself that by avoiding Johnson he could have the truth the way he wanted it.

But the truth would not cooperate.

One morning John came late to the breakfast table. He sat down, caught his breath and began to cough hard as if trying to dislodge something from his throat. He swallowed a couple of times and shook his head. "I'm sorry, Mom," he said weakly. "I don't have time to eat. Could I just have some real hot tea?"

Polly put the kettle on the stove. As the water heated she sat down at the table. Her son looked wan, overtired. "John," she asked, "do you have a cold? You're terribly hoarse."

He nodded. "I think so. My throat's sore and I've got one of those damned eyeball headaches." He put his hand above his left eye and rubbed firmly. "I took some aspirin. I think they'll help."

They didn't. The hoarseness and headaches persisted. More disturbing to Polly, for the first time since his illness began John was losing his appetite.

Monday morning, December 22, was the start of Christmas vacation. Baker slept late. At mid-morning he rose and went to the bathroom. After brushing his teeth he leaned low over the basin to rinse his mouth with water cupped in his hands. All at once, like a blow from a white-hot sledgehammer, a blinding pain struck him in the temple just above his left eye. He staggered back against the wall and clutched a towel rack to keep from falling. All around him the room was spinning crazily. After agonizing minutes the whirling room slowed down. He pulled himself to a corner, braced his feet and put both hands to the sides of his head. He pressed hard against his temples. The buzzsaw in his brain ground to a stop. The pain ebbed, but his legs were rubber.

He stumbled back to his room and threw himself across the bed. He lay there without sleeping for two more hours.

At noon he felt steady enough to rise and dress. He went to the kitchen just as Polly came in from the back yard. "I thought I heard you stirring," she said. She went to the sink and started washing her hands. "Shall I fix you some brunch?"

He shook his head. He opened the refrigerator and poured himself a glass of orange juice. "This is all I want."

He drained the glass in a couple of gulps and set it on the sink next to his mother. "Mom, I think I'll go see Doctor Johnson." Then he left the house.

Doctor Johnson laid the test results across the top of his desk and studied them. He had ordered the tests immediately after John had revealed his symptoms earlier that afternoon. Now, as he had so often before, John sat in the brown leather chair near-by.

Johnson swiveled his chair around and looked at the X-rays clipped to the backlight. At last he flipped off a switch and turned back around facing John.

"John, the malignancy has spread upward from your chest. There's a nodule in your throat, and . . ."

"And it means another operation," John said grimly.

Johnson shook his head. His countenance was solemn. "No, John. The tumor has reached your brain."

As though it were a reflex, John jerked his hand to his left temple. "And that's the reason for the headaches—for what happened this morning in the bathroom?"

147

Johnson nodded. "I'm afraid so."

John lowered his hand and looked up at the ceiling. He swallowed hard a couple of times and began to shake his head slowly from side to side.

Johnson started to get out of his chair. "Are you all right, John?"

John lowered his head. His eyes were brimful with tears he was trying to hold back. He nodded. "It's just that . . . I thought I had a chance." After a moment he added, "I guess I've been fooling myself."

Johnson looked again at the papers on his desk. He waited for John to regain his composure, then looked up. "John, you say you've been having these headaches for over two weeks. Are you taking any medicines I don't know about?"

John shook his head. "Just aspirin."

Johnson was puzzled. He believed John, yet something was wrong. Johnson pointed to the test results. "All the evidence in these tests tell me that you've had some pretty painful moments, perhaps even intense pain." He leaned forward so that he could study his patient's reaction. "Aspirin won't make a dent in pain like that. You must have been doing something else."

"Just ignoring it," John replied.

Johnson asked, "How can you ignore it?"

For the first time John revealed the antidote for pain he had developed in the hospital following his second operation. "To be truthful, Doctor, I haven't known a moment without pain since that day. But I can control it."

Johnson was flabbergasted, but now the answers to questions that had bothered him for months began to fall in place. John had developed intense powers of concentration

148

to defeat other runners. Now he was using them to cope with pain. Through sheer force of will he had turned the tables on the odds. He was still functioning in a demanding job and meeting life head-on at a stage in his illness when, statistically, many others would already have succumbed to hopelessness. It was the most remarkable example of willful perseverance Johnson had encountered.

Impressed, Johnson said, "John, what you've just told me is extraordinary. But we must face reality. I'm going to order intensified radiation and chemotherapy for you. But that won't alleviate your pain." He looked at John kindly. "John, your time is almost here. There's no need for you to suffer unnecessarily. There are medicines that will help you."

"You mean sedation—shots?"

"If need be," Johnson replied.

"And they'll put me on a high, like the one I was on in the hospital?"

"That's one of the side effects, yes."

John considered the offer for only a few moments. Then, speaking slowly, he said, "Doctor, I thought for a while that I might luck out of this rap. But, today . . . well, I guess I'm going to die young." He took a deep breath and exhaled slowly. "OK. I'm not afraid of death. But I've got a lot of things yet I want to do for my kids. And I've got to be fully responsive to them, not hyped up." He shook his head. "No shots, for now."

Without argument Johnson nodded. "I understand, John. We'll delay sedation just as long as possible."

Johnson pushed away from his desk and leaned back in his chair. "John, there's something I've been wanting to say to you for some time. Not as your doctor. But as one

149

man to another. I've never mentioned this to you, but at one time in my life I wanted very much to be a professional coach. If it hadn't been for medicine, I'm sure that's what I'd be today, doing the same thing you are, working with young children. So, I've got a feeling for what you're accomplishing as a teacher. Lately, I've become even more aware of your work on a personal basis. As you probably know, I have a son in the fifth grade at Aspen."

"Bruce," John said.

Johnson nodded. "Yes, Bruce. You know, he never took any interest in track—competitive running—before. But in the year he's been with you he's changed. He eats, sleeps and breathes track. He practices at all hours on the mesa near our home. And he can't wait for your classes to start. Your influence on him has been nothing but good. And I'm grateful to you for that. But there's another reason for telling you all this.

"John, the sad fact is that you will probably never see the results of the wonderful things you're doing. But I want you to know—and I think I'm in a good position to make this judgment—that you've done more good in this world in your twenty-five years than most people who live three times that long. And you've done it where it will pay the biggest dividends, with youth. I've always felt the quality of a person's life is every bit as important as the quantity. On that score, John, you will outlive us all."

Deeply moved by the unexpected tribute John could not respond.

Johnson sensed his embarrassment. "Well," Johnson said, rising from his chair, "that's enough sermonizing." He stepped around his desk and put his hand on John's shoulder. "Don't forget this talk, John, or that I'm available to you at any time."

"I won't, Doctor. And . . . thanks."

As soon as John had left his office, Johnson leaned across his desk and pushed his intercom. "Liz, would you step in here a moment please?"

He was standing in front of his bookcase when his receptionist rapped on the open door. Pulling a volume from the shelf and sitting back down at his desk, he said, "Liz, that's one of the most unselfish men I've ever known."

"Mr. Baker? Oh, yes sir. I've heard about his work at Aspen."

Johnson nodded. "I'm sure. Liz, I need about thirty minutes of privacy. Can we make it?"

"Yes, sir. I'll take care of it. Just buzz when you're ready for calls."

For the next fifteen minutes Johnson studied the test results again, searching for any clue for hope. He found none. Then, picking up the desk phone in front of him he pushed the intercom. "Liz, I want to talk to these people in whatever order you can reach them." He gave his receptionist the names of four prominent urologists at two universities and two major hospitals in New York, Washington and Los Angeles.

For the next thirty minutes he picked the brains of his distant colleagues, probing for any newly developed surgical procedure, any new treatment, that might help him prolong the life of John Baker. Each of his colleagues assured him the treatment he had prescribed for his patient was all that could be done. They also confirmed what he already knew—it wouldn't be enough.

151

Wm. J. Buchanan

Distressed, he hung up the phone and pushed it away. He noticed his hand was trembling. The discovery startled him. He sat back in his chair and forced himself to relax. He was falling into a trap physicians must avoid. He was becoming emotional about a patient.

Chapter 13

The beginning of 1970 arrived in Albuquerque with characteristic southwestern capriciousness. Despite the calendar, the city basked beneath sunny skies. Only the dormant trees and off-green lawns bore witness to the season.

On Sunday, January 25, the temperature soared above sixty. Bored by the weekend that kept him from his work at Aspen, John filled the restless hours that afternoon in the driveway in front of his home washing and waxing his Triumph. Laboriously, he attacked each square inch of the tiny car's body, buffing and rebuffing the blue-green enamel to a brilliant sheen. For the dozenth time in an hour he stepped back to admire the results.

"You can do this one if you ever finish that one!" someone called from the street.

At the sound of the familiar voice, John turned around.

Parked at the curb, at the wheel of his parents' car, was John Haaland.

Baker smiled. "How long have you been there?"

"Long enough to know you've got more energy than sense," Haaland replied. "Come here and help me out of this thing."

Haaland swung his still-weakened left leg out of the car and reached back across the seat for a pair of crutches. "Thank God for automatic shifts," he said.

Baker helped him to his feet. Adjusting the crutches under his arms Haaland swung himself forward, landed on his good right foot, thrust the crutches ahead again and repeated the practiced maneuver until he had crossed the Bakers' front yard in a half-dozen giant strides. Baker ran ahead, moved a heavy wooden lawn chair from the porch and helped Haaland settle his lanky frame in it with his mending leg resting on the ground in front of him.

"How come you didn't ride your bike over?" Baker asked with a wry smile. He was fully aware his friend's motorcycle was a mangled pile of metal in his garage.

"Rub it in all you want," Haaland retorted. "But I promise you, I'll be riding that bike again before summer's over. And it'll be as good as new." He dropped his hand. "Besides, you'd better be good to me. This isn't a social call. I'm here to make you a proposition."

Baker sat down on the ground in front of Haaland and leaned back against one of the large elms. "What sort of proposition?"

Haaland's manner became more serious. "John, do you remember the Duke City Dashers?"

"Sure," Baker replied.

The Dashers were a track team for girls from first grade

154

through highschool that had broken off from another team called the Olympettes a few years earlier.

"Well, they've had a rough time of it, trying to make it on their own," Haaland said. "Then, Tony Sandoval took them over. He's trying to put the club back on its feet. Tony came to see me yesterday. He's got some great ideas for the Dashers. But he can't do it all himself. He needs help—and a lot more well-trained runners."

Haaland shifted in the hard chair to ease the burden on his leg.

"You've got some fine girl athletes at Aspen," Haaland continued. "So have I, at Zuni. Now—here comes the proposition—what if we combined forces with Tony? Each of us concentrating on his own specialty and recruiting runners from his own school, and any others who want to participate?" He added enthusiastically, "John, I honestly believe we could forge the Dashers into a real power."

Baker looked surprised. "You mean co-coaches? You, Tony and me?"

"That's right," Haaland replied. "It would take plenty of work and lots of time. But I know we can do it."

Baker leaned back against the tree. He stared through the barren branches toward the cloudless sky. Still holding the cheesecloth he'd been using for a buffer, he absentmindedly wrapped the rag tightly around his hand, unwrapped it, then wrapped it tightly again. After a while he asked, "John, have you really thought this through? I mean, the work I don't mind. But I don't know about . . . a lot of time."

Haaland shook his head impatiently. "There's no more thinking to do. Tony wants you. So do I. If this thing is to work we need you. So do the Dashers."

"The Duke City Dashers," John said, wistfully lingering over the words. "I like that." He burst into a wide smile, jumped to his feet, and stuck out his hand. "Johnnie my boy, for better or worse, you've just recruited yourself a coach."

Once again John had countered ominous news about his worsening condition by shouldering another burden. To his duties as full-time coach at Aspen, to his self-imposed extra-curricular chores as manager of the Aspen Early-Bird Clinic, he added the role of co-coach of the Duke City Dashers.

The Dashers' training schedule was time-consuming. Four afternoons a week after school, and often on weekends, the fifty-four teen-age and sub-teen members gathered with their new coaches at one of Albuquerque's city parks or in the rugged Sandia foothills to practice for hours the full range of AAU-endorsed track and field events.

For the first week Baker just observed the practice sessions. What he saw was what he had expected. Coming as they had from the playing fields of over a dozen different schools, the girls were a mixed lot, both athletically and in their attitudes. By studying the girls' approach to training, John could guess the kind of coach each had trained under. Most were level-headed, with an eager-to-learn approach to the Duke City Dasher way of doing things. But there were a few John thought he could help: the girls who had been trained under coaches who treated female athletes as a joke; the girls who had been treated as "stars" and extensions of their coach's own ego; the girls who had been taught that the greatest sin was losing; and, saddest of all to John, the girls who had been browbeaten for their imperfections. He decided to ensure two things: (1) every Duke City Dasher, from the swiftest to the slowest, would have equal status with her teammates and (2) membership in the club would be fun.

One favorite Dasher practice area was Roosevelt Park in the southeast section of Albuquerque. The large park provided enough open space to accommodate all the Dashers' routines, yet had many protective trees to shade the girls during rest periods.

One afternoon, following a vigorous practice session, John Haaland called the Dashers together at one corner of the park. "OK," Haaland told the assembled girls. "One last lap around the park before we call it a day."

A chorus of anguished cries filled the air. A couple of the fourteen-year-olds grasped their chests theatrically and dropped to the ground. "Oh crud, Coach," one Dasher complained loudly. "We're all wrung out." Immediately the other girls took up the chorus.

In the midst of the brouhaha Baker walked up beside Haaland and raised his hand for quiet. "All right," he said. "Pipe down and I'll make you a deal. Every girl who finishes one last lap around the park gets a double-dip ice cream cone—on the coaches."

In a twinkling the two prostrate girls leaped to their feet and took off around the park in a spirited jog. In short order every Dasher was following close behind.

"Old buddy, do you realize just how many ice cream cones it's going to take to pay off that gang?" Haaland said.

"Sure," Baker responded wryly. "One apiece." The following week, on Saturday, Baker showed up at Roosevelt Park driving his father's Oldsmobile. He parked near some pine trees and walked over to where the Dashers were pre-

157

paring for afternoon practice. As he drew near, Haaland nodded toward the Oldsmobile. "Did that sardine can of yours finally blow up?"

Baker smiled a noncommittal smile.

Three hours later, sweat-soaked and bone-tired, the Dashers finished their final laps and dropped to the ground with moans of exhaustion. Baker let them rest a few minutes, then blew his whistle for attention. "OK, Dashers. You see that brown car over there under those trees? There's a surprise waiting there for any girl who makes it from here to there in a homestretch sprint."

In one bobbing mass the Dashers, with Baker running in their midst, sprinted across the park to the trees. Baker gathered them around the rear of the car, bringing the six- and seven-year-olds to the front so they could see better. Then, he unlocked the trunk of the car and threw the lid open. The trunk was loaded with cold watermelons.

"Hey, Coach," one of the older girls asked. "Where'd you get those this time of year?"

Baker grinned. "That's my secret."

For the next half-hour the Duke City Dashers gorged themselves on melons that Baker had arranged for a friend to bring up from Mexico.

As the Dashers grew in their skills other Baker-catered rewards followed. One week there was soda pop and chips; another week, Polly's homemade ice cream and cookies. One Saturday a bell-clanging pizza truck arrived at the park and served the bug-eyed Dashers hot pizza slices and cold lemonade. Soon, all over town, girls who had never expressed any interest in athletics began badgering their parents for permission to try out for "the fun club"—the Duke City Dashers.

Soon after joining forces, Sandoval, Haaland and Baker decided it was time for the Dashers to have an official uniform. For days the three young coaches worked over sketches. At last a consensus was reached. The Dashers would compete in dark green shorts and jerseys bordered with yellow piping and the initials D.C.D. across the chest. A matching green warm-up suit completed the outfit.

On uniform preview day the Dashers lined up at Roosevelt Park while proud parents snapped hundreds of photographs. Standing near the edge of the crowd, beaming, Baker turned to an equally pleased John Haaland. "You know," Baker said, "I'm really proud of our 'little green machine,'" The nickname stuck.

The first public intramural event for the newly reorganized and growing Dashers was held one weekday afternoon after school, in late March, in the rugged Sandia foothills east of Albuquerque. Eager to display their skills to friends and parents, the girls had worked for days organizing a variety of track and field events, competing against each other. The events were staged by four different age groups: 9 and under; 10 through 11; 12 through 13; and 14 and older.

As always at foothill events a dedicated crowd of nearly two hundred fifty track fans watched from open truck beds, from atop cars and campers, or beneath large patio umbrellas staked like giant multicolored mushrooms along all sides of the staging area. To complete the carnival atmosphere, teenage entrepreneurs strolled among the spectators hawking hotdogs and cold soda pop. As the games progressed, the applause and cheering of the fans spurred the Dashers to spirited performances.

The final race of the day was a one-mile cross-country by members of the 12-to-13 age group. Five girls were participating. One, twelve-year-old Jeanne Kroker, had just recently joined the Dashers.

At the gun the five pushed off from their starting crouch in a fast pace. But the rough dusty track soon took its toll and the gaps between them widened. In the lead two of the fleetest Dashers maintained a neck-and-neck sprint. Strung out far behind, the three others struggled along.

Packed along both sides of the homestretch, the spectators cheered on the two neck-and-neck runners. But ignoring the shouting around him, John Baker stepped back from the crowd, shaded his eyes, and looked at the last runner just topping a final hillcrest before entering the homestretch. It was Jeanne Kroker. John could see the girl was crying.

A half-minute later, doggedly fighting to remain on her feet, Jeanne crossed the finish line last and collapsed onto the ground in a torrent of tears.

John was at her side at once. Gently he put his arm around her. At his touch she looked up. "Oh, Coach," she sobbed. "I tried. I really tried. But I just couldn't do it." She buried her blonde head deep against his arm.

He put his hand beneath her chin, tilted her head up and touched her lips with his finger to still her crying. Then, lifting her to her feet, he held her close and smiled down at her. "Jeanne, you did your best, and you kept running. You didn't quit. You have nothing at all to be ashamed of." He squeezed her tightly. "Honey, I'm so proud of you. You ran a magnificent race!"

160

Through her tears Jeanne stared at John in awe. All around her others were congratulating the winners. Yet he, her coach, was congratulating her, even though she had come in last! Impulsively, she wiped her tears on the sleeve of his jacket and smiled.

"There," John said. "Now you're all pretty again. Go get into your warm-up suit before you catch cold."

From a low hillside overlooking the staging area, where he had set up his cameras to capture photos of the Dashers in action, Ray Kroker had witnessed the whole scene. As his daughter had stumbled toward the finish line he had deserted his equipment and rushed down the hill to intercept her. Her coach had gotten to her first. Now, as Jeanne ran toward him, Kroker saw that his daughter was smiling.

Jeanne rushed up to her father and grabbed his hand. Breathlessly, she told him what John had said to her. "He's proud of me, Daddy!" Still beaming from ear to ear, she broke away and rushed off happily to find her warm-up suit.

Touched, Kroker scanned the crowd for John, determined to thank him for his attention to Jeanne. But John wasn't in sight. Suddenly remembering his unguarded equipment, Kroker started back up the hill. He made a mental note to call John that night.

Near the crest of the hill, Kroker retrieved his cameras and tripods and slipped them into their cases. As he did he looked back toward the track area. The crowd was beginning to disperse. But something else caught his eye. Off to one side, behind a boulder where he couldn't be seen, was Coach Baker. Kroker watched him curiously. He was doubled over with his hands tightly clutching at his abdomen. He was retching violently.

For a moment Kroker thought of going to John's aid.

161

Then, thinking his presence might be more embarrassment than help, he decided against it. After all, he thought, with all the excitement of the afternoon, it was probably nothing more than a nervous stomach.

That evening, and on many evenings that followed during which they became close friends, Ray Kroker did, indeed, thank John Baker. But the scene behind the rock was forgotten, until months later.

By the end of spring the Duke City Dashers was a club to reckon with. Throughout the southwest at meet after meet the finely honed team began to make its mark in track circles as it scored victories over unsuspecting rivals. Despite his penchant for de-emphasizing winning as a prime goal of children's sports, no one was more pleased with the growing Dasher reputation than John.

To help recruit promising talent for the club, he enlisted Chuck Lander and Ron Jones. They haunted the playing fields of schools throughout the city scouting likely candidates for Coach Baker's "Green Machine."

On Saturday afternoon, April 11, 1970, the Duke City Dashers hosted an Invitational Track Meet at John's old arena, University Stadium in Albuquerque. At the edge of the field, accompanied by Chuck and Ron, John shouted encouragement as the Dashers put on a sterling performance. Toward the end of the meet, John turned to his two young friends and said enthusiastically, "Fellows, we're on our way. The Dashers are going to the National AAU finals. And they're going to bring home the championship!"

From a nearby bench, a gruff voice called out, "Hey, John you've been standing in the sun too long, pardner."

John turned to see a local radio and television sports announcer grinning at him. They were good friends. The

162

sportscaster had once chronicled John's own track feats. With a flourish John raised two fingers in a V-for-victory sign and flashed a smile. "I meant every word!" he called back to the scoffer.

It was a heady prediction for such a young club. But, unabashed, John repeated it widely.

Seven months later, Carlos Salazar, Sports Editor of the Albuquerque *Tribune*, would recall John's bold prophecy in print. The Duke City Dashers would remember it too.

Chapter 14

Throughout that spring of 1970, under the watchful eyes of Sandoval, Haaland and Baker, the fledgling Duke City Dashers continued to upgrade their athletic skills. In deference to the unpredictability of the springtime weather the girls came to practice each day prepared to work out in shorts and jerseys or in the more cumbersome, but protective, warm-up suits.

One March afternoon at Roosevelt Park the sunny skies quickly turned overcast. As always on the high desert plateau the sun-blotting clouds were accompanied by plummeting temperatures. In minutes the thermometer dropped to the low forties. A steady north wind compounded the chill.

At Sandoval's signal the Dashers donned their warm-up suits for a first run around the park perimeter. At their side, dressed in his UNM Lobo jacket, John joined the exercise.

165

Wm. J. Buchanan

At the far end of the park, near the site of the watermelon feast, John stopped when he noticed a small girl huddled up in a patch of pine trees. Wearing a light-weight shirt and denim jeans, she was inadequately dressed for the change in weather. Hunkered down into a tight ball, her knees pulled close to her chest, she was shivering.

John waved the Dashers on. Changing course, he ran over and knelt down beside her. She greeted him with a faint blue-lipped smile.

"Hi!" John said. "I bet you feel like an icecube."

The girl nodded with a convulsive shiver.

"Here," John said, "let me show you a game I used to play with my father when I was little." He unzipped his jacket quickly and pulled the girl close to him. "This game is called 'toast and toaster.' You're a piece of bread and I'm putting you in the toaster to make you crispy warm." He pulled the zipper shut, enclosing the chilled girl inside against the warmth of his chest with only her head protruding from the top of the jacket. "See," he said. "Now you're a piece of toast and I'm a big old toaster."

The little girl felt much better.

Holding her tightly, John rose and jogged across the park to the Dasher staging area. He picked up a loose warm-up jacket from a pile of clothing, freed the girl and put the jacket around her snugly. Then he sat on the ground beside her and hugged her close. On the field the Dashers were practicing sprints. The little girl was watching with interest.

"What's your name, honey?" John asked.

The girl didn't respond.

He tapped her shoulder and repeated the question. As he

166

did he realized the girl's eyes were riveted to his mouth. She was reading his lips!

"Stephanie," the girl replied. Then, pointing toward the field, she said proudly, "My sister's a Dasher!"

John nodded. Beneath Stephanie's bobbed, light-brown hair her tiny face sparkled as she followed every movement of the Dashers. John tapped her shoulder again. "How old are you, Stephanie?"

Stephanie held up four fingers.

John smiled. "You know, pretty soon you can be a Dasher, too."

Stephanie's face clouded over. She shook her head. "I can't," she said solemnly.

"Can't," he chided. "Now, what do you mean by that?"

Reaching down with her small hands, Stephanie pulled up her right pants leg. From her knee to her ankle the leg was supported by a lightweight brace.

John was startled. Although he'd carried the girl across the park in his arms he hadn't noticed the brace.

At four o'clock a pale-green Datsun pickup truck pulled to the curb where the Dashers were just ending their final routines. Still huddled next to John, Stephanie pointed to the truck and shouted, "There's my momma!" At the same moment, seven-year-old Lori Keel left the field where she had been practicing and ran over to Stephanie. She reached out her hand to her little sister. "Momma's here, Stephanie."

Stephanie started to rise. John reached over, lifted her, and sat her astraddle his neck. "I'll give you a piggy-back ride." With Lori running at his side he jogged off across the the park holding the delighted Stephanie on his shoulders.

At the truck John put Stephanie in the front seat. Lori slid in beside her. Seated at the wheel, Lois Keel smiled at her daughters, then at John. "It looks like you've been babysitting, Coach. Thanks."

"It was a pleasure," John responded. "By the way, Mrs. Keel, we've been going over some summer schedules we want to get the parents' comments on as soon as possible. I have a copy over at my gear. I wonder if you have a minute to step over and take a look?"

"Certainly," Mrs. Keel agreed. "You girls wait here."

He led her across the park to where the Dasher equipment was lying. He leaned down and picked up a clipboard. Pointing to a blank page on the board he said cryptically, "This is for the girls' benefit if they're watching."

"Oh?" Mrs. Keel said, puzzled.

John took a deep breath. "Mrs. Keel, I hope you won't think I'm overstepping. But, I saw that Stephanie is wearing a brace. And . . well . . . I wonder if you'd mind telling me what's wrong?"

Without hesitation Mrs. Keel shook her head. "Not at all. Stephanie has chronic osteomyelitis."

"Osteomyelitis?" John considered the term for a moment.

"That's a bone disease, isn't it?"

Mrs. Keel nodded. Yes."

They talked for fifteen minutes. With deepening interest John listened to all Mrs. Keel could tell him about her daughter's affliction. The infectious disease, most common to children, had already caused a sharp deterioration in Stephanie's hearing. Now it was attacking her leg. The latest report from Doctor Rakestraw, Stephanie's physician, was heartbreaking. Unless Stephanie overcame her reluctance

168

to therapy, she was in danger of being permanently crippled. It was even possible that she could lose her leg.

"What kind of therapy, Mrs. Keel?" John asked.

"She's supposed to lift a heavy sandbag, tied to her foot, several times a day. But it's too painful to her. Getting her to do it is just plain torture. Steve—that's my husband—and I have tried everything. But Stephanie's just too young to understand how serious it is."

He thanked her for confiding in him and walked her back to her truck. As the truck drove away, Stephanie leaned out the window and waved. With a smile, John waved back.

At dinner that evening John picked at his food. His preoccupied silence set his parents on edge. Finally, her concern overcoming her discretion, Polly asked "John, is there something your father and I should know?"

"I'm sorry," John responded. "I'm OK. Really. It's just something that happened today at practice." In detail he told his father and mother about his encounter with Stephanie Keel and what he'd learned about the child's illness from her mother.

"It's cruel," he said, shaking his head. "She's only four years old."

Jack and Polly glanced at each other. Each knew instinctively what was on the other's mind. Their son was dying. Yet, instead of indulging in self-pity he seemed more concerned about a crippled child. They had never been prouder of him than they were at that moment.

After a while Polly said, "Surely there's something someone could do."

"You know," John said after a thoughtful moment, "I think so too." He stood and pushed his chair under the table. "Don't wait up for me. I might be late getting home."

169

The night librarian at the UNM Medical School Library looked up at the wall clock, then glanced again at the engrossed young man hunched over a stack of books at a corner table. He showed no signs of leaving. The librarian sighed. She didn't want to disturb him. But rules were rules.

"Sir, I'm sorry, but we must close now."

Absorbed in the open book before him, John Baker didn't respond.

"Sir!"

With a start, John looked up, surprised to see the young lady standing beside the table. He glanced at his watch. It was ten minutes after eleven. "Good lord," he said. "I didn't realize it was this late." The librarian smiled at him. "That's all right. But we are supposed to close at eleven."

He grabbed his notes. He was seated at the same table where ten months before he had done research in books on urology to discover for himself the fatal course of his advanced cancer. But this time the books before him were on bone diseases; specifically, osteomyelitis.

He stuffed his notes into his pocket and returned the librarian's smile. "Thanks," he said and hurried out the door.

There was no need for him to refer to the notes. Of the information he had gleaned on the crippling, bone-deforming disease of osteomyelitis, one paragraph on therapy had almost jumped off the page at him. But did the remedy apply in Stephanie's case? He was determined to find out.

The heavyset gray-haired lady behind the reception desk at St. Joseph's Hospital shook her head again. "I'm sorry, sir," she said adamantly, "but Doctor Rakestraw simply cannot be disturbed now. He's on rounds and won't be finished for at least another hour."

John looked at his watch in frustration. "But I have classes then. Can't you just page him and let me speak to him a minute on the phone?"

"That's out of the question during rounds, except in case of emergency."

With a sigh of resignation John half-turned from the desk. "All right," he said. "What ward will he be coming down from?"

"Three," the receptionist replied, and immediately regretted it. Like a shot John turned and bounded up the steps across the lobby.

"Sir!" the hapless receptionist called after him. "That's against the . . ."

It was too late. John was already out of sight.

At the top of the second stairwell, he pushed open a heavy swinging door and entered a large corridor. All around him was the hubbub of a busy hospital. Warily he looked up and down the hallway. At a nurses' station a few feet away a group of white-coated men stood in conference. Could Doctor Rakestraw be in that group? John wondered. It dawned on him he had no inkling what Rakestraw looked like. He walked up to the group and smiled. "Doctor Rakestraw?" he said pleasantly.

A middled-aged, slightly balding man turned and peered over his glasses curiously. "Yes?"

Boldly, John put his hand on Rakestraw's shoulder and nudged him to one side away from his colleagues. "Doctor," John said, speaking fast, "my name is John Baker. I'm a teacher as Aspen Elementary School. I also coach a

171

local girls' track team. There's a sick child—one of your patients—that I must talk to you about."

Rakestraw was taken aback. Then, intrigued by this determined young man, he led John by the arm into a near-by stockroom. "All right, young man. What's on your mind? But make it fast."

Hastily John described what he knew about Stephanie, including the information he had picked up the previous evening at the medical-school library. After five minutes he finished talking.

To Rakestraw there was something captivating about the brash young man. His sincerity was apparent. "You say you've talked to Mrs. Keel already?" Rakestraw asked.

"Yes, sir," John replied. "She said you could call her if you want."

Rakestraw shook his head. "No, that won't be necessary. I'm sure it's perfectly all right." He stepped toward the door. "I've got to continue my rounds. Come along. We can talk on the way."

They walked side by side. "You've certainly given yourself a good capsule understanding of the case," Rakestraw said. "I only wish some of my university students were as talented at research. But, to your essential question: Stephanie, I fear, is one of those cases where the child responds well initially—the drugs managed to arrest the progress of the disease—but doesn't respond well to therapy. It's a long painful physical process, and with children as young as she is it's often difficult for them to really understand the necessity for all that hurting."

John was barely able to stem his excitement. "Then what I read *does* apply to Stephanie. I mean, running could be beneficial to her."

Doctor Rakestraw stopped at the doorway of a patient's room. "I really don't know," he said. "But in a situation where she's motivated enough, involved enough . . . " He looked at John and smiled. "Sugar-coated medicine!" he said. "You know—now don't expect miracles—but it just might help."

John grabbed Rakestraw's hand and pumped it enthusiastically. "That's all I wanted to hear, Doctor. Thanks."

He turned and started at a fast walk down the corridor.

"Hey!" Rakestraw called after him. "Keep me informed."

"I will, Doctor," John called back over his shoulder. "And thanks again."

During lunch break that noon John went to the Aspen administration office and looked in the phone book for Steve Keel's number. Mrs. Keel answered the ring. "Mrs. Keel, John Baker. I wonder if you could arrange to have Stephanie show up at Dasher practice this afternoon? Don't tell her I asked you to bring her."

"Sure, Coach Baker. I'll bring her along with Lori."

At two-thirty that afternoon Stephanie hopped down from her mother's pickup truck and limped across Roosevelt Park toward where the Dashers were limbering up. John ran over and took her by the hand. He led her back to the staging area and whistled for a huddle of all the Dashers. As the girls gathered around him he motioned for silence. "Dashers," he said, "there's someone here today who has been one of our most enthusiastic supporters — Stephanie Keel. This afternoon we're going to honor her with a special recognition."

As Stephanie and all the girls watched in anticipation, John reached into a sack at his side and pulled out a small

173

green Dasher jersey. Ceremoniously, he put the jersey over Stephanie's head and slipped it down over her body. "Stephanie Keel," he intoned in an official voice, "by the authority invested in me as coach I hereby name you an honorary Duke City Dasher!"

Stephanie's face lit up and she grabbed the front of the jersey with both hands and pulled it out from her so she could see it better. All around her the Dashers whistled and applauded their approval.

John raised his hand again. "Now, there are rules that go with this appointment."

The Dashers grew quiet.

"One," John said, "every new girl who joins the Dashers will have to race first against Stephanie."

The Dashers laughed and applauded.

". . . and two; at every practice session the top three girls in any category will have to race against Stephanie."

Again the Dashers shouted their approval.

Gleefully, Stephanie entered into the spirit of her new status. At her first race that afternoon the small girl crouched down at the starting line, prepared to sprint against two new Dashers. At the gun the older girls darted away. Stephanie remained in her starting crouch.

While everyone stared, puzzled, John ran to Stephanie's side. Silently, he chastised himself for not thinking of this problem before. He knelt down beside Stephanie and tapped her on the shoulder. "Stephanie . . . watch." He pointed toward John Haaland and motioned for him to fire the starting gun again. As Haaland pulled the trigger a puff of blue-white smoke billowed out the end of the barrel. John pointed toward the smoke, then turned Stephanie's head toward him. "When you see that puff of smoke—run!"

The little girl nodded. From that point on no opponent ever got a headstart on Stephanie.

Her progress was slow. At first she could only run a few yards. Gradually, as the practice sessions went by, her distance increased, foot by agonizing foot.

One afternoon during a hearty sprint Stephanie suddenly collapsed and clutched her right leg at the knee. Biting her bottom lip she began to cry. "It hurts! It hurts!"

John was at her side at once. He scooped her up in his arms and carried her to the sidelines. He looked her leg over carefully. Then, he put his fingers to both sides of his mouth, stretched his cheeks, bugged his eyes and contorted his face into a grotesque shape. "BOOLA! BOOLA! BOOLA!" he chanted loudly.

Stephanie stopped crying and asked, "What's that for, Coach?"

John made another ugly face. "THESE—ARE—MONSTER—FACES!" he intoned slowly and solemnly, "TO—SCARE—THE—PAIN—AWAY!"

Stephanie laughed. So did John. "All right," he said. "Now, you make one."

She stuck her fingers into her mouth and pulled her cheeks askew. "Boogie—Boogie—Boogie," she said, trying to copy John's fierce chant.

"Is it working?" he whispered.

With her fingers still in her mouth Stephanie looked down at her leg. "Uh huh," she said with a solemn nod.

"Good," he said. Then, in hushed tones, he added, "Now remember, whenever mean-old-man pain tries to grab hold of your leg, you just keep making these monster faces to scare him away. OK?"

"I'll remember," she said seriously, "I promise."

175

At subsequent races when Stephanie would suddenly puff her cheeks and bug her eyes into a horrid mask while running, bystanders would stare dumbfounded. But to John, smiling knowingly on the sidelines, it was the most beautiful face in the world.

Years later, in February 1973, in a special awards ceremony in Albuquerque, Stephanie Keel proudly marched to the dais to receive the first-place medal for a one-mile cross-country race. It was one of many medals to come. In the audience, Doctor Rakestraw turned to Lois Keel. Deeply moved by the occasion, Rakestraw told her that without question John Baker had saved her daughter from a lifetime in a wheelchair.

Chapter 15

By force of will John made it through the school year at Aspen without sedation. But by mid-summer the pain that now attacked every fiber of his body could no longer be ignored. Still uncomplaining to family and friends, John admitted to himself that the day was near when he would have to ask Doctor Johnson for sedatives. Characteristically, he kept putting that day off until it was no longer a matter of his choice.

Late Friday evening, July 17,1970, John busied himself in his bedroom putting the finishing touches to a list of race schedules for the next day. Saturday the Duke City Dashers were competing in the Junior Olympic Track and Field Championship Meet at University Stadium in Albuquerque. It was a major event for the Dashers and one John had been looking forward to for months.

As he sat working at his desk he accidentally pushed

some papers onto the floor. He reached down to pick them up. Suddenly an excruciating pain struck him in his lower right back. He stood up, grasped at his back with both hands and wheeled toward the door. Before he could take a step, his knees buckled. He fell to the floor in a kneeling position beside his bed. Fearing he might fall sideways and be unable to get up, he threw his upper body across the bed, stretched his hands over his head, and clutched at the bedspread. Growing in intensity the searing pain suffused his abdomen, then crept up through his chest, neck and head. He opened his mouth to cry out. Instead, he clamped his teeth over his bottom lip and bit down. *I must not scream,* he told himself repeatedly. Incredibly, his worst fear at that moment was that if his parents learned of his condition they would try to stop him from going to the Dasher meet the next day.

Calling on his last strength he pulled himself onto the bed and rolled over on his back. Clutching a pillow he moved it near his head, stuffed a corner of it into his mouth and bit down hard. Then, squeezing the headboard tightly, he prayed for the blinding agony to stop. *Just for tomorrow's meet, he begged . . . just one more day!*

At 8:30 Saturday morning Polly rapped on her son's bedroom door. He was scheduled to leave at 9:00 and should have been up and finished with breakfast by now. There was no response to her knock. Slowly, Polly pushed open the door and looked inside. "Oh, my God, no!" she cried aloud.

Drenched in a pool of sweat, deathly pale, John lay on his bed staring up at his mother. At the sides of his mouth trickles of blood oozed from his discolored, swollen lower lip where he had bitten through the flesh to keep from crying out. The bedspread and sheet were knotted in a tangled mess, mute evidence that he had thrashed about in pain throughout the night.

Polly rushed to her bedroom phone and dialed Doctor Johnson's office. For seemingly endless seconds she waited anxiously for the ring. "I must not panic," she kept reminding herself aloud. "I'm all alone. It's up to me."

Doctor Johnson's receptionist listened to Polly's hurried explanations.

"Mrs. Baker," the receptionist replied, "Doctor Johnson won't be back in town for several days. I realize that John must have forgotten to mention this to you. But Doctor Kagey is taking our calls. Please hold on."

Within seconds Doctor Herman Kagey was on the line. Once again Polly quickly described her son's condition.

"Mrs. Baker," Doctor Kagey said, "I want John taken to the hospital at once. Do you want me to arrange for an ambulance?"

Polly knew she could drive to Presbyterian Hospital in seven minutes at most. Fearful of the added minutes an ambulance might take, she decided to take the chance. "No, Doctor. I'll bring him myself."

She rushed back to the bedroom. "John," she asked sharply, "can you walk at all?"

"I'll try," he said weakly.

With a strength unknown before Polly pulled her son to his feet, draped his arm over her shoulder and half-carried, half-dragged him through the house, across the yard, and put him in the back seat of her car. Leaving her home wide open, she jumped behind the wheel and sped down Louisiana Street to the Freeway. She was at the emergency-room door of Presbyterian Hospital in five minutes.

179

The double room just across the hall from the Ward Three nurses' station was empty. Working with speed, Nurse Jane Woltz and an orderly lifted John from the wheelchair and put him onto the bed nearest the door. Beside the bed a tall portable I.V. stand was already in place. Hanging from the stand, dangling above John's head, the medication ordered by Doctor Kagey immediately after Polly's call was ready to be administered.

With things apparently under control, Polly left the room and stepped down the hall to call Jack. At John's side Nurse Woltz began to charge the I.V. needle in preparation for inserting it into John's vein. Then she stopped and looked around the room.

"Tom," she said to the orderly, "quick, get me a restraining board and some tie-down tubing."

The orderly left the room.

On the bed John had curled all at once into a fetal position. "Oh-h-h!" he cried out in agony.

Dropping the needle, Nurse Woltz grasped his arms and rolled him over onto his back. At her touch John opened his eyes and stared blankly. Suddenly, out of his mind with pain, he put both of his hands flat against her chest and shoved with all his might. "DAMN IT, KEEP AWAY FROM ME!" he screamed.

Propelled by the force Nurse Woltz fell backward over the adjacent bed. At the same time John grabbed the I.V. stand and sent it flying across the room. It struck the far wall but didn't break.

Terrified and in tears Nurse Woltz fled the room, seeking help.

Gasping for breath John fell back on the bed. Fitfully, he rolled from side to side, moaning and crying.

Then, strong arms pinned him at the shoulders. "John, lie still!"

The voice sounded familiar. Still unable to see, John tried vainly to focus his eyes. "Doctor Johnson?" Like a child in desperate need, he grasped the arms that were restraining him and held on tightly.

Standing above John, Doctor Kagey opened his mouth to correct his patient. Then, thinking better of it, he let the illusion stand. He put his hand on John's brow. "John," he said. "I'm going to give you a sedative. It will stop the pain. Do you understand?"

At the sound of the voice he thought was Johnson's, John lay still. "Yes," he moaned. "Yes . . . it's time."

Ten minutes later he was in a deep, sedated, painless sleep.

Tests showed that the malignant tumor had firmly re-entrenched itself in John's abdomen and was now threatening his kidneys. With no alternative, Doctor Kagey ordered the most intensive chemotherapy treatments John had yet received. Ten times, over the next two weeks, John's arm was strapped to a rigid restraining board while massive doses of chemical antibiotics were injected into his bloodstream to combat the marauding cancer. Each treatment took six hours.

For the first forty-eight hours John lingered on the threshold of death. Then, slowly, almost miraculously, he began to rally.

On the third moring he opened his eyes to find a young, attractive brunette nurse taking his pulse. She smiled at him. "Hi," she said. "I'm Jane Woltz. How are you feeling?"

"OK, I guess," he said weakly. "But you'll have to excuse me for not rising. Something you're putting into me has left me like a marshmallow.''

"Well," she said, "that's a lot safer for me than when you first came in.''

John arched his eyebrows. "Oh, oh," he said. "One of the night nurses told me about that. Are you really the one?''

She nodded. "I'm the one.''

Embarrassed, John flushed. "I don't know what to say.''

She smiled. "You don't have to say anything. I understand." She took her hand from his wrist and made a notation on his chart. "You're doing much better.''

Glad that the young woman had forgiven him, he smiled back. "Thanks," he said.

"Don't mention it. Oh, by the way, Doctor Kagey left orders to put you in a private room. But there're none available right now. And I'm afraid you're going to get a roommate after a while. A fifteen-year-old boy. He was in a hang glider accident—clobbered by a tree from what I hear. It looks like he might lose an eye. Anyway, if it gets too uptight for you, let me know, and we'll try to work something out.''

"He lost an eye?" John said.

"Looks that way. Now, remember what I said.''

He nodded. "Sure," he said. But his thoughts were already on someone else.

He awakened to strident voices. He glanced at his clock. It was mid-afternoon. The curtain between the two beds was drawn. On the far side of the curtain, a woman's voice was pleading. "Jimmy, they did all they could. But the eye was just too badly damaged." The woman's voice choked into a sob. "I tried to warn you. You just wouldn't listen."

"Oh, Mom," a younger voice cut in angrily, "cut the bitching, will you? I'm the one they butchered. I wanted to be a pilot. Now look at me. All I'm ever going to be is a freak!"

Throughout the night and the next day the boy's self-pitying tirades unsettled his family, his doctor and the ward nurses. His mood seemed to swing wildly between two poles. When not loudly complaining against fate, he would lie for hours staring glumly out the window, refusing to communicate with anyone.

The day after the boy's arrival Polly listened to him with mounting anger. *How much she would give,* she thought, *to be able to trade her own son's affliction for a lost eye!*

John sensed her ire. Calmly, he reached over and placed his hand on top of hers. "Mom," he said, "when you come back tonight I want you to bring me something from my room." He told her what he wanted.

"What on earth for?" she asked.

He smiled. "Just bring it. OK?"

At nine o'clock that night, after evening visiting hours were over, John picked up the book his mother had brought him. Holding it open at a preselected page he carefully stepped out of bed and pushed back the curtain that separated him from his roommate.

Jimmy was sitting up in bed morosely staring out the window at the city lights glowing in the valley below the hospital. At the sound of the curtain sliding back he turned to John. One side of the boy's face was covered with a heavy padded bandage.

183

"Hey," the boy said, surprised. "What're you doing?"

John smiled. "I've got something to show you, Jimmy."

The boy's jaw set. "I don't want to see anything," he said caustically.

Still smiling, John said, "Well, you're going to, whether you want to or not." He laid the open book on Jimmy's lap.

Taken aback, something told Jimmy his so far silent roommate should be listened to. He looked down at the book. It was open to a full-page picture of a man dressed in boots and a leather jacket with a white scarf wrapped loosely around his neck. The man stood by an open-cockpit airplane. He was wearing a patch over his left eye.

Jimmy reached down and picked up the book. "Who's that?"

"That," John replied, "is Wiley Post. Ever hear of him?"

"No."

"Well, you should have. He was one of the most famous aviators in history. He won all sorts of trophies for flying. He was the first man ever to fly around the world alone. And," John added pointedly, "he did it with only one eye." Beginning to feel increased pain, John stepped back to his bed and sat down. "And having only one eye never stopped him from doing what he wanted to do. Or lots of other famous people either. And there's something else about those eye patches, too."

Now interested, Jimmy asked, "What?"

"They add an air of mystery," John said. "It drives women wild. They just can't resist a man like that."

Jimmy slapped his leg hard and grinned. "Hey, wonder how I'd look in one of those things!"

"Let's find out." John reached over to his bedside table

184

and picked up a strip of purple ribbon Polly had also brought at his request. He tied the ribbon at a rakish angle around Jimmy's head and fixed it in front where it looked as if it were part of the boy's bandage. "A real one will be smaller. But this will give you an idea. Look in the mirror."

With a bound from bed Jimmy rushed over to the mirror, turning from side to side, studying his image from all angles as he strutted proudly before the mirror.

At visiting hours next afternoon Jimmy's mother stopped just inside the doorway and stared in disbelief. Seated at his bedside Jimmy and his roommate were playing a spirited game of checkers.

"Jimmy," the surprised mother said, "why is that ribbon around your head?"

At the sound of his mother's voice Jimmy jumped up and started preening again in front of the mirror. "How about this, Mom?" he said proudly. "It's an eye patch. It's deb-on-airre-e-e! Mr. Baker told me about them. He knows a lot about things like that." Jimmy grinned. "But he doesn't know much about checkers. I've already beat him three times."

With a loud harumph, John cleared his throat.

Jimmy smiled. "OK," he said. "Three games out of seven."

Next morning in the patients' lounge at the end of the ward, Jane Woltz sat down at the table where John was sipping a cup of hot tea. She said appreciatively, "Everyone's talking about how much Jimmy's changed, John. How in the world did you manage it?"

John shrugged. "I don't know, Jane. I guess it's all a matter of finding the right button."

* * *

As his strength gradually returned, John became impatient to get back to coaching the Dashers. But the treatments had to be continued, under hospital scrutiny, for several more days. John decided to make the best of the long stay. He had his mother bring him some clothes and his cassette-tape player from home and started roaming the hospital corridors in cut-off jeans and a T-shirt, playing his favorite recordings for all who would listen.

One afternoon at the nurses' station he came upon Jane Woltz in conversation with an attentive young intern. Jane smiled and called John over. "John, I want you to meet Ernie, my fiancé."

They chatted amicably for several minutes. Then John turned to leave, but quickly he turned back to the couple. "By the way, Jane," he said, "when you get ready to give me that special massage—you know," he winked suggestively, "I'll be in my room."

With a crafty smile he walked away, leaving the tongue-tied girl and her discomfited fiancé staring blankly at each other.

Despite his pranks John's stock on the ward was high. Each day a bevy of doctors, nurses and patients, many old fans of the once champion miler, dropped by his room to visit. Soon, visitors to the ward learned that John's condition could be judged by the general mood. When he was down, the ward glumly reflected his suffering. When he rallied the ward mirrored it. All who came in contact with him were affected by his spirit and charm.

Saturday morning, July 25, Polly walked with her son to the patients' lounge and helped him fix his tea. At the table she pulled an envelope from her purse, looked at it a few seconds, then reluctantly handed it to John. "This came this morning," she said. "I didn't know whether to bring it or not."

He opened the envelope. It contained his teaching contract for the 1970–71 school year at Aspen.

Anxiously, Polly watched him study the document. Then, he reached across the table. "Let me borrow your pen."

With exaggerated strokes he signed his name to the contract, folded it and handed it back to his mother. He asked her to mail it at once. "Mom," he said with determination, "when Aspen opens this fall I'm going to be there, coaching."

On August 3rd, sixteen days from the day he entered Presbyterian Hospital near death, he was released. As he packed his clothes Jane stepped into his room. "John," she said, "Mr. Barber across the hall would like to see you before you go."

From the propped-up bed in a private room a frail, elderly man beckoned him to his side. From earlier chats John knew that Barber was seventy-nine years old.

The old man smiled wanly and stuck out a thin, trembling hand. John took his hand and held it.

"John," the old man said, "I just want to thank you for all the visits you paid me—and for that pretty music. It was kind of you. Mighty kind."

"Mr. Barber, it was a real pleasure talking with you. I enjoyed our visits very much."

The old man squeezed John's hand. "Let me tell you something, John," he said with an air of ancient wisdom, "enjoy your youth. When you get to be my age you'll find it ain't no great shakes."

Without changing expression John nodded. "Yes, sir,

187

Mr. Barber. I'll remember that. And thanks." He bade the old man goodbye and left.

Once home, John was almost immediately plagued by a new problem. He couldn't keep food down. With mounting alarm Polly tried a variety of diets—juices, ices, gelatins, purees. None worked. Steadily, John weakened.

Desperately, Polly pleaded with her son to re-enter the hospital. "They can feed you intravenously until we find something you can eat. But this way, you're starving!"

He refused. His mother was right, he knew. He was, literally, starving. Grimly he recalled a fact from the books at the UNM Medical School Library. Many cancer patients, he remembered reading, succumb prematurely to malnutrition. He was determined it wouldn't happen to him.

He began to experiment with food. Day and night he haunted the family kitchen, concocting recipes.

One morning he cried out loudly, "Mom, come here!"

In the back yard pruning roses, Polly dropped her shears and rushed into the house. At the kitchen table, with an obviously just-used dinner plate in front of him, John sat staring at the wall clock. "It's been nearly an hour!" he exclaimed.

The meal stayed down.

As excited as a scientist who had just made a revolutionary breakthrough, he explained to his mother what had happened. He had eaten a bland meal of milk-toast. Immediately, he had to rush to the bathroom to throw up. In a fit of anger he had stalked back to the kitchen, slapped together a monstrous sandwich of cheese, baloney, lettuce, onion, pickle and mustard and wolfed it down defiantly. It hadn't made him ill.

188

"The only thing I did differently," he said, "was eat right after I threw up."

That afternoon he repeated the experiment. As expected, the first meal came up at once. But the second, eaten immediately afterwards, stayed down.

On the spot, mother and son made a pact. At all hours of the day or night when John got hungry, Polly fixed him two meals.

"Just make sure," he chided his mother, "that the first one is left-overs."

Chapter 16

In spite of his continuing show of good humor to his family and friends, as summer passed, John began to experience a new ailment, one he had never faced before. It was a sickness of the spirit.

Since January, when he joined the Duke City Dashers, he had given up Sunday church services. "I'm not worried about my soul," he had explained at the time to his parents, "but I do need every hour I can find to work with my kids."

Now, as his body grew noticeably weaker with each passing day, he began to doubt the existence of a God who would exact such a harsh penalty from one who had tried to do His will. As his faith waned, he turned toward the occult.

Like all major universities, the University of New Mexico had attracted its share of iconoclasts who sought the answers to mankind's eternal questions through esoteric studies. As a student John had known professors who unofficially spearheaded such study groups. With tolerant amusement he had considered them, and the students they attracted, as eccentrics. Now, uncharacteristically, he sought them out. Increasingly, after work, he spent his time on the UNM campus attending metaphysical seminars. Late one evening in August, following one seminar, he came home in a wrought-up mood and slumped onto the couch.

Jack had gone to bed, but Polly was still up. She asked, "What's the matter, John?"

"I'm going to change doctors," he said. His voice was tense.

"But why?" Polly asked.

"Because all those damned chemicals and rads they've been dosing me up with are poisoning me. That's why."

Polly tried to conceal her alarm. "Who told you that, John?"

He mentioned the name of a doctor she'd never heard of. He wasn't a local physician, but traveled extensively, speaking mostly at or near universities.

"I've talked with him twice. Tonight we had a long session alone. He's cured a lot of cancer patients by teaching them to take control of their own lives, to concentrate on their inner healing power. He teaches how to purge your mind of distracting concepts—religion, love, even family—and make *yourself* number one. Think of it. My mind can cure my body!"

Wisely, Polly realized this was not the time to try to argue it out. She knew he was grasping at straws. But she had to do something.

The next morning, after a sleepless night, she made an appointment with Reverend James Hawk.

Sixty years old, slight with reddish-brown hair and a happy nature, the Reverend Hawk was minister of education at Central United Methodist Church in Albuquerque. Though not the pastoral minister, he was known for his sympathetic understanding and willingness to hear any problem at any time, day or night. His compassion and availability had made him a busy and highly regarded counselor in the largest Protestant congregation in New Mexico.

Reverend Hawk had talked with Polly before about her son, and he was worried about her. Now, as he listened to her again this afternoon in his office, his worries were not assuaged. She was speaking of John's deteriorating condition, and of his "grasping at straws." As always, she sat ramrod straight, bravely smiling as if she were discussing her next choir solo.

Instinctively, Reverend Hawk knew that this devoted mother was suffering as much, if not more, than her son.

"I was wondering," Polly concluded, "if you could help."

"Why?" Reverend Hawk asked.

Polly was startled. She looked at him questioningly.

He looked straight at her. "I mean that. Why? Look how strong you are, how easy it is for you to sit here and talk to me about your dying son. Do you really need my help, or anyone's? Aren't you capable of bearing this burden all by yourself—without me, or your family, or your friends?"

It was as if she had been struck a blow. Her face flushed and her lips began to tremble. Then, in frustration and despair, her voice almost a whimper, she said, "Oh, my God . . . no-o-o," and collapsed in her chair sobbing.

He let her cry until her tears would no longer come. Then he stepped around his desk and took her gently by the arm.

He led her to a couch and sat down beside her. "I'm truly sorry, Polly," he said. "but I've felt for a long time that that was necessary."

She looked up and saw his eyes were red.

She poured out her heart to him, her anguish, her feelings of helplessness, her fear that her son was now turning against his faith. "Is there anything you can do . . . anything at all you can say to him?" she pleaded.

Reverend Hawk was silent for a long while. Then he said, "There might be. You go home and let me take the burden for a while."

As the conflict within him grew John began to spend the late hours following the UNM seminars at the clubs and taverns he'd enjoyed in happier days—the Territorial House, the Sidewinder, the Wine Cellar. One night he asked Dianna Briggs to go with him to Corrales.

They had been together often in the year since they had renewed their friendship at the Sidewinder Tavern. In time, John had found in her presence a sustaining comfort, and she became his confidante. To her he revealed his most cherished dreams—both past and present.

This night at the Territorial House he told Dianna about his newfound philosophy and his plans to give up conventional medical treatments.

From the look on her face he could tell she didn't approve. His mood soured. He yelled across the room at the waitress and ordered another margarita.

"John," Dianna said, "you're drinking too much."

"Oh God," he said bitterly "not you too. I'm so sick of all of you. Hovering over me. God, if I could just get away to die in peace." He downed the remainder of his margarita in one gulp. "Do you know that I've always lived at home, Dianna. Except for a year in California, and a couple of months when Haaland and I rented a get-away apartment. That's pretty damned sad, isn't it? Twenty-five years old and never my own man."

He yelled at the waitress again and asked what was holding up his order.

"John," Dianna said. "I want to go home."

"What are you talking about? We just got here."

"Take me home, please."

He was angry. He threw some bills on the table and stood up. "Come on." He walked toward the door and she followed behind, running to keep up.

He started the Triumph, then looked across the river to Sandia Peak. "You know. I almost drove off there once, in this car, right after I learned I had cancer. Sometimes I wish to God I had."

Dianna didn't say a word.

He gunned the engine and roared out of the parking lot, throwing gravel. For the entire wild half-hour ride to Dianna's home, they said nothing.

He pulled into her driveway, left the motor running and sat waiting for her to get out. She turned to him and said, "I don't know what's changed you, John. I don't know you this way. And I don't want to be a part of it. But I'm going to pray for you."

She jumped out of the car and ran to the house.

He drove around aimlessly, then noticed with surprise that he was on the university campus. He parked at Tappy Hall, walked across the street to Pine and Copper Avenue and entered the sanctuary of Central United Methodist Church, where he had worshipped since childhood; where,

195

at fifteen, he had been voted the outstanding youth of the
year. Alone in the deepening twilight, he sat on a rear
bench, staring at the high altar, pondering the imponderable.

On succeeding days, compelled by an urgency he
couldn't understand, he returned repeatedly to the church,
always in the evening when the sanctuary was empty.

One evening as he sat in the darkening church he heard
someone softly call his name. Startled, he looked toward
the aisle. The familiar figure of his educational minister was
standing there.

John started to get up. "Reverend Hawk!" he said. "You
surprised me."

Reverend Hawk put out a hand and motioned to John to
remain seated. "Sit down, John, please. I didn't mean to
disturb you. Do you mind if I sit with you a while?"

"Please do," John replied.

Reverend Hawk sat down beside John on the cushioned
hardwood bench. "I've seen you in here several times recently, John. I wonder if I can be of some service to you?"

John looked at the pleasantly smiling older man for a long
time. He had always admired Reverend Hawk. Good-
humored, indefatigable, the reverend was noted for his
ability to counsel people of all ages and all walks of life, as
equals, both to him and in the eyes of God. With a twinge of
nostalgia, John recalled that it was to Reverend Hawk that
he had first revealed his plans to marry Mary Ann.

"Reverend Hawk, I've got terminal cancer. I'm almost at
the end."

With a barely perceptible nod Reverend Hawk replied
softly, "I know, John."

John's eyes widened. "You know?"

"Please try to understand, John," Reverend Hawk said evenly. "But your mother has been in need of solace too."

Somehow the thought of his mother seeking the understanding comfort of this good man pleased John deeply.

"I'm glad of that," he said sincerely.

He was silent a long time. Then, turning in his seat toward Reverend Hawk, he said. "But I don't understand things anymore, Reverend. I try. God, how I try. But it just won't make sense for me. I've tried to do what's right. Oh, I'm no saint—I don't want to give that impression. but I don't think I deserve this . . . this hell." He shook his head bitterly. "Why, for God's sake?" he asked, looking at Reverend Hawk beseechingly. "Why?" he repeated in anguish.

Reverend Hawk didn't reply.

John leaned back against the bench and stared at the high altar. After a moment he said plaintively, "I know you can't answer that." He breathed a deep sigh. "I couldn't expect you to know what it's like. It's impossible for me to explain, or for anyone to understand."

After a moment Reverend Hawk said evenly, "I'm dying too, John."

The words stunned John. Was he mocking him? No—not James Hawk.

Calmly, Reverend Hawk nodded. "I've got advanced lymphoma. A lymph tumor. You've probably heard of it as Hodgkin's disease. I've been in pain for a long time, and have to go to the hospital regularly for treatment. That's all that keeps me alive. But it's too far along. I'll never beat it."

John was overcome with self-recrimination. *How could he have been so stupid,* he agonized, *so self-pityingly selfish*

197

to have fallen into the trap of thinking his suffering, his anguish, was unique? His body began to shake. "My God!" he said, as tears filled his eyes. "My God!" No other words would come. Without lowering his head he looked squarely into James Hawk's eyes and wept openly.

They remained there for hours, discussing their lives, their fears, their mutual deep-rooted conviction of the immortality of the soul. Late that evening they reached a special agreement. From that night on, at least one evening a week, John and Reverend Hawk met in the sanctuary of their church to pray for their own and each other's souls. It was the end of John's doubts, and the beginning of a deeper, sustaining friendship between two benevolent men that lasted until October 22, 1970, when suddenly, and without warning, James Hawk died.

Polly broke the news to John gently. "Do you want to go to the funeral, John?"

He shook his head. Nauseated from one of the treatments Reverend Hawk had urged him to continue, he said, "I'm going to avoid funerals . . . just as long as I can."

Chapter 17

Sustained now by massive sedation which he took orally every hour, but refusing to let the cancer rule his life, John returned to Aspen in the fall of 1970, as he had vowed.

Weak in body, but strong in spirit, he soon devised a scheme to keep himself close to his children. Unable to participate for long in their games, after the first few minutes of each play period he would retire to a sideline bench. There, like a field marshal directing his lieutenants, he would coordinate all play through his loyal student aides— Chuck Lander, Bill Witherspoon, Anthony Straquadine and, on the frequent occasions when he dropped by, Ron Jones.

One day as the bell rang for the end of outside activity, Bill Witherspoon ran up and sat down on the bench next to John. The boy looked up apprehensively. "Coach," he said, "I'm afraid I let you down."

"Oh," John replied. "Now how did you do that?"

"My mom's a nurse," Bill said. "I told her about
. . . last year. When I helped you get dressed, and how
God-awful you looked." Bill's face mirrored his anguish.
"Are you mad at me?"

John shook his head. "No, I'm not mad at you. What did
your mother say?"

"She was worried. She talked to some people at her hospital, where she works. I didn't know she was going to do
that. But, anyway, later she told me I should watch you real
close, here at school. And that if you ever got sick I should
go tell someone in the office. Is that right?"

There was a long silence. After a while John put his arm
around the boy's shoulder. "Bill, your mother just might be
wiser than I was. Don't be upset with her. And, yes, if you
ever see me sick, and I can't talk to you, go and tell Mrs.
Mercer at once. OK?"

Relieved but still concerned, Bill nodded. "OK."

Each afternoon after school and on weekends when the
Duke City Dashers held practice sessions John continued to
coach his beloved "green machine." By now the Dashers'
ranks had swelled to over one hundred members, plus three
additional coaches. The steady growth of the club, coupled
with the Dashers' continuing good showing at track meets,
pleased John enormously. Yet, as he had the previous year
at Aspen, he sensed that tangible rewards for the girls were
lacking.

One afternoon he showed up at Roosevelt Park carrying
a shoebox. Mysteriously holding the box high above his
head, he blew his whistle for a huddle. The Dashers gathered around him quickly.

Grinning with boyish delight at the attention his scene

was creating, he opened the box with flair and held its contents aloft. In his hands two highly polished gold trophy cups shone in the afternoon sun.

"Sally"—he motioned toward one of the girls—"would you step up here, please."

With a puzzled smile, a thirteen-year-old freckle-faced girl with long brown pig-tails stepped forward. Anticipating John's purpose, the rest of the Dashers broke into applause. Sally was the finest all-around athlete in the club.

John handed Sally one of the gold cups. "For you, Sally," he said, "for setting a wonderful goal for all the rest of us to shoot for."

The Dashers applauded.

Holding the second cup high he looked out over the bobbing heads. The Dashers waited eagerly.

He spotted the girl he was looking for. "Alice"—he motioned toward the girl—"come here, please."

A murmur of surprises rippled through the assembled Dashers. From the rear of the group a twelve-year-old blonde with a long pony-tail held with rubber bands stepped forward timidly. She had never won a race, had never even finished well enough to get her name mentioned in the Dasher re-cap bulletins.

With a flourish John placed the second cup in the amazed girl's hands. "For you, Alice," he said grandly, "for never giving up. For always trying. For showing us all what true courage is."

For one frozen second the Duke City Dashers stood silent. Then, as the lesson of the gesture they had just witnessed sank in, they erupted in an ovation of whistles and applause, gallantly and wholeheartedly endorsing the award.

201

As the Dashers returned to practice, John Haaland walked up to Baker's side. "John," Haaland said, "that was beautiful. But where did you get those expensive cups?"

With a friendly shrug, Baker left the query unanswered.

From that day on, for the rest of his time with the club, John selectively awarded gold and silver trophy cups to deserving Dashers—winners and tryers alike. No one questioned his source again.

One morning a few weeks later, Polly switched off the vacuum cleaner in her son's bedroom and sat down on the edge of his bed. Something was out of place. She returned to her cleaning chores, still vaguely dissatisfied. Picking up her dust rag she cleaned his desk, his chair, his bookcase. . . .

His bookcase!

With a start she stepped back and looked at the bookcase. John's trophies had been rearranged. But that wasn't all. Several were missing.

She started to leave the room to phone John at work, but then remembered something she had heard about him giving trophies to Dashers. She knew at once what had happened to his trophies. Her eyes misted over. With a feeling of awe, respect, and love for her son she realized the trophies he had been awarding were his, with his own name burnished away.

Soon after school opened that year, John began an unusual but meaningful routine. After Dasher practice every afternoon, instead of going home, he drove directly to the home of one of his students. Well-known by all the parents, he was welcomed everywhere as family. Often asked to remain for dinner, he would sit at the table but would seldom eat. Taking only a cup of tea or sometimes a glass of milk he would decline other food, explaining, falsely, that he had eaten a late lunch.

The calls were not social. Driven now by a compulsion to make every moment count, he made his visits with a purpose. At each home he steered the converstion to the children. He told the parents everything he had learned about their children's hopes, talents, and needs. He didn't hesitate to mention his own feelings about how each child's needs could best be met. Often during a single evening he would call on three or four families. Not one resented his involvement in their family affairs.

One evening, during a visit to Doctor Johnson's rambling home in the Sandia foothills, John glimpsed a regulation-size billiard table in Johnson's game room. With an air of nostalgia he walked over to the table and ran his hand slowly across the green felt covering.

"Do you play?" Johnson asked.

Sensing a challenge, the man who had been noted as having one of the best billiard eyes at the University of New Mexico replied guardedly, "Oh, some."

"How about a game?"

John could barely mask his enthusiasm. "Well, I'll try."

An hour later, chagrined and unsmiling, he hung up his cue. He had been soundly defeated!

With a wry smile, Johnson, not unaware of John's poolroom reputation, gave his friend a patronizing pat on the back. "Better luck next time, Champ."

John shook his head dispiritedly. "I think I've been hustled."

The two good friends laughed.

Ten days later, during a routine check-up in Johnson's

office, John brought up the still rankling defeat. "How about a rematch!" he asked.

"Any time," Johnson replied.

The following Saturday afternoon John soundly defeated Johnson three out of three games on Johnson's home turf. Amazed at John's masterful performance, Johnson hung up his cue. "I just don't understand it," he said.

It was John's turn to gloat. "No hard feelings, Doc. I was just off the last time."

Years later, by chance, Doctor Johnson learned that during the interval between those two friendly but spirited matches, John, still fiercely competitive, had taken night lessons from a professional billiard player for the sole purpose of defeating Johnson in the last match John ever played.

Tuesday evenings Jack worked late at his downtown office and ate dinner before coming home. Polly and John dined together. Late Tuesday afternoon, September 22, Polly answered her kitchen phone. "Mom," John's voice came over the line, "have you put dinner on yet?"

"I'm just getting ready to. Why?"

"Put it back in the fridge," he said. "I've got to go on a shopping spree. Meet me on the mall at Coronado Center around five-thirty and I'll treat you to a steak."

Polly was already loosening her apron. "It's a date," she said.

She got to the mall precisely on time. Her son was sitting on a shaded bench near a giant water fountain in the plaza of the huge shopping center. He hadn't seen her approach. She paused a moment and watched him. He had his legs crossed casually, his left foot resting on his right knee. Propped against his thigh was an open hard-bound ledger.

Oblivious to the passing crowd, he was absorbed with writing in the ledger.

Polly walked up to the bench. "Hi," she said.

With a start John closed the ledger and shoved it back into a paper sack bearing the logo of a local department store. Sack in hand, he stood up and greeted his mother.

Polly glanced around. There were no other packages. She nodded toward the sack. "Is that your 'shopping spree'?"

He grinned sheepishly. "That's it. Hey, are you hungry?"

"That, I am," Polly replied.

He escorted her across the mall to a popular restaurant. Just inside the foyer the hostess stepped up and called him by name. "This way, Mr. Baker."

The hostess led them to a table on the far side of the dining room next to a sliding glass door that opened out onto a shrub-lined patio. Polly understood the choice of table at once. Her son had arranged for this particular table, in advance, so that he could leave the room immediately if he became ill.

He ordered a light meal and ate cautiously. Then, after the first few bites, he smiled. Polly was glad to see the smile; it was his way of saying he was going to be all right.

They ate slowly, lingering over each course, purposely protracting this precious time between them. All too soon, it was over. As John picked up the check, Polly reached across the table and put her hand over his. "John," she said with great feeling, "thank you for the most beautiful evening of my life."

He didn't reply. This, they both knew, would be their last outing.

*   *   *

Wm. J. Buchanan

By the beginning of October, too weak now to stand for long periods, John spent most of his time at Aspen or at Dasher practice, sitting on the ground, shouting instructions to his pupils. To his family and closest friends his deteriorating condition was dramatic. He was thinner, with a noticeable gauntness in his face. Yet, his spirit was so upbeat that even at this late stage few others suspected the seriousness of his illness.

One who knew the truth was John Haaland. And, as the crisp fall days passed, Baker revealed to his best friend a deepening fear that plagued him now more than any other.

They were sitting side by side at Roosevelt Park, watching the Dashers go through their routines. After a while Baker turned to Haaland, "John, you'll be starting cross-country training in the foothills soon. I'm afraid this is where I get off."

"What do you mean?" Haaland said.

"Look at me," Baker replied ruefully. "I can't even walk across this park without sitting down to rest. What good would I be to the Dashers in the foothills?"

Haaland said angrily, "John, as long as you can sit up, hear thunder and see lightning you're essential to this club. Now cut out the defeatist talk. We'll find a way."

Though it was not fully understood, John's worry about possibly having to leave the Dashers spread through the club. Two afternoons later, as John sat on the sidelines at Dasher practice, he saw the Keels' pickup truck pull up to the curb next to Roosevelt Park. As Lori and Stephanie scrambled out John saw their mother wasn't driving, This time the girls' father had brought them to practice.

Steve Keel stepped out of the truck and walked with his

daughters across the park. As the girls broke away to run to where the Dashers were assembling, Keel continued over to where John was sitting. He smiled down at John, then, without fanfare, pointed to the curb and said, "John, do you see that green Datsun sitting over there?"

John nodded.

"Well," Keel continued, "every afternoon after school either me or my wife is going to be sitting in that truck outside your office at Aspen. And we're going to take you and whatever equipment you want to tote along to wherever the Dashers are practicing. And we're going to get you back to your car, or home, afterwards. No ifs, ands or buts about it. Understand?"

Touched, John tried to respond. "I don't know . . . what can I say?"

"You can say, 'yes!' " Keel said insistently.

John nodded. "Yes," he said hoarsely.

From then on, each afternoon the Dashers practiced, Steve or Lois Keel would meet John at Aspen, load his gear, and head for the training area in the Sandia foothills. At the training ground they would gun the little Datsun up a steep incline to the top of a low hill that sat in the center of the area. There they helped John spread blankets and cushions over a large flat boulder. Settling himself on the rock, he would don a huge Mexican sombrero one of the Dashers had made specially for him. For the rest of the afternoon, like a king on his throne, he would shout instructions to his beloved Dashers as they sweated through their practice routines on the field below.

Friday afternoon, October 9, from his seat atop the hill, John saw the Dashers suddenly break ranks and mob

207

around Haaland. The huddle was too far away for him to hear what was going on. All at once the assembled Dashers let go with a loud "HOORAY!"

From the midst of the group one of the girls broke into a run up the hill toward John. As she drew near, he saw that it was Kathy Kroker, Jeanne's nine-year-old sister.

"Hey, Coach!" Kathy yelled at the top of her lungs. "It's come true! It's come true!"

The exhilarated girl stopped just short of his perch and fought to catch her breath. He stepped down from the rock and put his hands on her shoulders. "What, Kathy?" he asked, almost as excited as she, "What's come true?"

Kathy took a deep breath. Then, beaming hugely, she blurted, "Your prediction! We just heard. The Dashers are going to the National AAU finals in Saint Louis next month!"

Unable to remain standing, John sat back against the large rock. Slowly, his eyes filled with tears. Kathy's smile faded. "Coach, are you all right?"

He reached out and pulled the pert blonde girl to him and hugged her tightly. "Yes," he said. "Everything's fine, Kathy. Just fine."

The little Triumph sat parked at the edge of the Glenwood Hills overlook, high above the eastern fringes of Albuquerque. Far below, like millions of candles afloat on an ebony sea, the lights of the sprawling city glowed for miles in all directions. In the front seat, leaning with her back against the door, Dianna Briggs listened as John told her about the invitation to St. Louis.

"John, I'm so thrilled for you," she said. "What more could you ask?"

John replied, "To live long enough to go with them!"

He stared straight ahead into the darkness. "Dianna," he said after a long silence, "the dreams are done with now—the Olympics, a family of my own. I can accept that. God knows I don't want to die. But, if it must be, I can accept that too, as long as I can believe I'm leaving something in the world through these kids. But now, more than anything, my one last wish is just to live long enough to go with my girls to Saint Louis." Following their reconciliation after the explosive night in Corrales, John had increasingly unburdened himself to Dianna. And she had stoically played the role she knew he had cast for her in his mind. Outwardly detached, coolly unemotional, she had suppressed the instincts that welled up inside her to reach out and hold and comfort this gallant, suffering man. The pretense had taken its toll in tears after he had taken her home.

Now, on this night, she could no longer sustain her dispassionate image. As they talked, he had casually placed his arm along the back of her seat. His hand rested just above her shoulder. Suddenly, overcome by his fervid plea for life, she reached above her shoulder, grasped his hand and pressed it to her cheek. "John!" she said in anguish as her tears fell onto his palm. Impulsively, she put his hand to her lips and kissed it. "Oh, John!" she said again.

She felt his arm stiffen. Gently, he eased his hand from her grasp and took it from behind the seat. *Mother of God, no!* she thought. She knew that in one blind moment of pity and love she had blundered.

She sat up quickly, dabbed at her eyes with a handkerchief and forced a nervous smile. "Well," she said, trying to downplay the incident, "that was pretty stupid of me, wasn't it?"

Visibly tense, John switched on the dash light and glanced at his watch. "Hey! Do you realize what time it is? I'd better get you home."

They drove the ten miles to Dianna's home in silence. At the doorway of the big adobe house, she turned and looked at John beseechingly. "John, I'm so sorry."

He touched her lips with his finger. "Sh-h-h-h."

"You'll call again?"

"You bet." He bent down and kissed her tenderly on the cheek. "Thanks, Dianna. For everything."

She closed the door, rushed to the darkened living room and knelt on the couch in front of a large picture window. As she pulled back the drapes, the Triumph was just pulling out of the driveway. She watched the rear lights of the little car recede down the hill and fade into the night. "Goodbye, John," she whispered softly in the darkness. She knew she would never see him again.

Chapter 18

Saturday, October 24, John coached the Duke City Dashers in an Invitational Cross-Country Meet in Phoenix. He had been in severe pain when he left Albuquerque the day before, but he had once again hidden it from his parents.

As the meeting progressed, John sat on a bench near the finish line cheering the Dashers home. Nearby, several Dasher parents noticed that he was on edge. Moreover, every fifteen or twenty minutes he would take a small bottle from his pocket, fish out a pill and swallow it.

Standing with the group of parents, Lois Keel became disturbed as she saw John take a half-dozen pills in less than two hours. Nonchalantly, she moved toward the bench and sat down beside him. Within minutes he reached in his pocket and withdrew the bottle again.

"Coach," Mrs. Keel asked, "what's that you're taking?"

Without hesitation he showed her the label. She recognized the medicine at once. A barbituric compound, it was a powerful sedative. The recommended dosage on the label was one pill every two hours, as needed. There were two pills left in the bottle.

Mrs. Keel saw that John's mouth was white and drawn at the edges, and she became alarmed. "Coach, is there anything I can do for you?"

He nodded grimly. "Mrs. Keel, I've got to get to a drugstore."

The races were completed. The meet was beginning to break up. Mrs. Keel said, "I remember seeing a drugstore at your motel. We'll be there soon. Can you make it?"

He opened the pill bottle and swallowed the last two pills in one gulp. "Yes," he said, his voice strained. "But, please, let's go quickly."

Polly balanced the heavy bag of groceries in one arm and fumbled to get the key into the front door. She had heard the phone ringing since she had pulled into the driveway. Whoever was on the line was certainly persistent.

Finally getting the door open, Polly rushed to the kitchen, set down the bag and picked up the phone. "Polly Baker speaking."

"Ma'am, this is the long-distance operator in Phoenix, Arizona. I have a Mr. John Baker who wants to place an emergency call to Albuquerque and charge it to your number. Is that all right?"

"May I ask whom the call's going to?"

"A Doctor Edward Johnson."

"Yes," Polly said at once. "Put it through."

She placed the phone back in its cradle and sat down at

212

the kitchen table. She'd wait five minutes, she told herself. She stared at the kitchen clock. The minutes passed slowly. When she got Doctor Johnson's office his receptionist put him on the line immediately.

"Mrs. Baker," he said evenly, "I don't want you to become unduly alarmed. John was in need of medicine. He called from a drugstore, and I instructed the pharmacist on exactly what to do. John is coming home with a couple of Dasher parents. They're going to be driving through the night. I'd like to see him first thing tomorrow morning."

Shortly after dawn, Sunday morning, John lay on an examining table in Johnson's office while the doctor checked him. Though he had been heavily sedated and lying on the back seat, the 450-mile automobile trip had left him near total collapse.

While Johnson was checking his heart rhythm, John opened his eyes and said something too softly for Johnson to understand.

"I'm sorry, John, I didn't hear you." Johnson leaned closer to John's mouth.

John's voice was weak, barely audible. "Keep me alive . . . long enough . . . to go to Saint Louis."

213

Chapter 19

Oral medication no longer suppressed John's pain. Routinely, now, he had to submit to the Demerol injections he deplored. Still, doggedly, he held onto his jobs with the Duke City Dashers and at Aspen.

But time was running out.

Wednesday morning, October 28, he sat alone at his desk at Aspen waiting for the first outside play period to begin. Partially sedated, he was nevertheless experiencing great pain. But this pain was different. For the first time since the day he fell while running on the mesa, it was centered in his lower abdomen.

He sat back in his chair and raised his feet to his desktop. Closing his eyes he concentrated, trying to seize on some thought, some diversion, to drive this new hurting away.

The sudden jangle of the activities bell startled him. Feverish, beginning to shiver, he sat forward in his chair and took several deep breaths for control. He rose to his feet. Feeling faint, he grabbed the edge of the desk to steady his wobbly knees. In a few seconds the lightheadedness passed. He reached across his desk, picked up a football and walked out of his office into a brilliant, sunbaked October day.

The playground was already filled with children, running, climbing on equipment, chasing one another in spontaneous games.

John raised his whistle to his mouth. Surprised at the weakness of his breath he blew a feeble warble that was lost in the lively din. Shaking his head he walked into the middle of the romping children. "All right," he said, straining at the words, "let's get together . . . over here."

The faint-voiced command had no effect. Caught up in the headiness of unsupervised play, the children continued their roughhouse. A few feet away several kids were horsing around a water fountain, squirting one another.

Suddenly, enraged by the pain that was setting his pelvis aflame, John raised the football above his head. "SHUT UP!" he screamed at the top of his voice. "GET OVER HERE RIGHT NOW!"

With a violent downthrust of his arm he threw the football blindly across the playground. It sped straight for the terrified children by the fountain, grazing one girl's cheek. By ironic coincidence she was Tammy Johnson, Doctor Johnson's nine-year-old daughter.

All activity ceased.

For a few breathless seconds, rooted in pain. John looked at those young faces staring up at him in disbelief. Those faces! He had seen those looks once before. "Oh, no-o-o-o!" he wailed aloud as the reality of what he had just done struck him. His face turned white. With both hands he clutched at his abdomen. Grimacing in agony he collapsed onto the playground, rolled to one side and curled into a fetal ball. His body began to convulse. Fully conscious, he opened his mouth to speak, but words wouldn't come.

In the middle of the terrified children Bill Witherspoon had stood transfixed during John's tirade. Now, as his coach fell helpless to the ground, Bill ran to his side. As he knelt down, Bill's eyes locked onto John's for a telltale second. With a quick nod Bill jumped to his feet. "Hold on, Coach!" he pleaded. "I'm going to get Mrs. Mercer!"

Polly had just settled into her favorite chair for a short break from her household chores when the phone rang. She had taken this morning off from work and wondered if it was a call from her office. She picked up her cup of coffee and carried it to the kitchen. She lifted the phone. "Polly Baker speaking."

"Mrs. Baker, this is Veta Mercer. John has just fallen on the playground. He's in the nurse's office now. I think he should be taken to a hospital at once. But he absolutely refuses to let me call anyone but you."

Calmly, Polly set the cup of coffee she was still holding on the kitchen counter. "Tell John we'll be there in a few minutes."

She hung up the phone, waited a few seconds, then dialed Jack's number. "Jack. John's sick at Aspen. Come right home. I'll explain when you get here."

She hung up again, waited, then dialed Doctor Johnson's office and briefly explained the situation to his receptionist. "We'll have him there just as soon as possible," Polly said.

217

She sat down at the kitchen table. For a moment she debated calling Robert and Jill. She decided against it. It might not be *that* serious. She'd wait until she talked with Johnson. But in her heart she knew what she wouldn't let her mind admit. This was the beginning of the end.

Doctor Johnson finished taking John's pulse count and gently placed his arm back on the examining table. There was no question in Johnson's mind about what had caused John's collapse. He looked down at John. "Can you talk, John?"

"Yes." John's voice was weak.

Johnson pulled a stool to the head of the table and sat down. "The tumor has hemorrhaged. I'm afraid it might get worse. You've got to be hospitalized."

John turned his eyes to the ceiling. After a thoughtful silence he looked back at Johnson. "Tomorrow. OK?"

Johnson shook his head. "Today."

"Doctor. There's something I must do. Give me one day. I'll come to the hospital tomorrow. But . . . just this one day . . . please!"

Johnson was shaken. Torn between prudence and a strong sympathetic desire to let this valiant man live his last days as he wished, Johnson finally nodded. "John, your parents are right outside. I'm going to speak to them frankly. There are things we must watch for, every second. If any of them show up, I want you at the hospital immediately. Otherwise, I'll expect you there tomorrow."

With a pale smile John nodded. "Thanks, Doctor."

Polly awoke with a fitful start. She picked up her watch from the end-table. It was 8:00 A.M. Still weary, she pushed herself up and sat for a moment on the edge of the

218

couch, where she had spent the night, rising fitfully each hour to go to her son's room to check him during his deep sedated sleep. None of the signs Doctor Johnson had warned her against had occurred. After a while she got up and went into the kitchen. She would make the coffee extra strong this morning, she decided.

From the hallway came the sound of a doorway opening. Surprised, Polly stepped back into the living room. John was standing there, fully dressed.

"John! Where do you think you're going?"

"I'm going to school, Mom."

"School! But . . . that's impossible!"

With a soft smile he looked at her tenderly. "Mom, try to understand. There's something I have to do. I'll be home soon."

His manner left no doubt about his determination. Reluctantly, Polly stepped aside and watched him leave the house.

Kneeling near the corner of the cafeteria, Bill Witherspoon checked off several items of softball equipment just arrived that morning. Neither he nor the Aspen officials realized that several of the items had been ordered over and above allowances, and paid for secretly, by Coach Baker, from his personal funds.

As Bill hunched over the equipment he heard a familiar sound. He glanced toward the parking lot, just as John's little Triumph entered the Aspen campus.

Bill jumped to his feet, shouting, "Hey! Coach is here!"

The morning play session was in full swing. At Bill's yell all across the playground children abruptly stopped whatever they were doing and rushed to the south side of the campus, near the parking lot.

Without stopping, John drove straight through the parking lot and down the narrow alleyway beside the cafeteria. He parked as close as he could to the playground. As he got out of his car, he was mobbed by squealing and jumping children, all shouting questions at the same time.

Beaming, John walked over to a row of swings. The children gathered around him. He held up his hand for quiet. Then, resting against one of the metal upright anchor posts supporting the swings, he said, "I came back today, because I owe all of you an apology. Yesterday . . . what I did . . . was inexcusable." He paused and swallowed several times. Then, his voice choked with emotion, he continued. "I want you to know how sorry I am. I never did anything like that before. You all know that I love you . . . that I'd never intentionally hurt you. You . . . each of you . . . have meant more to me than you'll ever know."

He was weeping openly now. All around him children were crying too. He struggled to control his emotions. "This will be my last time here . . . with you . . ."

"No-o-o-o, Coach!" a chorus of voices rose in anguished protest.

"It's not because I want it that way," he continued. "It's just something that . . . I have no control over. Someday, you'll understand."

He paused and took several deep breaths. Then raising himself to his full height, he forced a smile. "Now, there's something you can all do for me. When you think of me in the future, don't remember me like I was yesterday, groveling in the dirt. Try to remember me like today, smiling with you, and . . . walking tall." He thrust out his hands. "Now, who wants to walk me back to my car?"

Immediately all the children gathered around him, grasping for his hands. For a full fifteen minutes he moved among them, stroking their cheeks, and patting their heads. At last, draping his arms over the shoulders of Tammy Johnson and Bill Witherspoon, and with all the rest of his children close to him, John Baker walked across the playing fields of Aspen for the last time.

Chapter 20

Hospital tests revealed that the seeping hemorrhage was disrupting John's heart rhythm. Struggling to compete with the rapidly metastasizing tumor, his heart took on a dull, metallic beat that was audible to people near him. To replace the lost blood Johnson ordered transfusions. John took five pints of whole blood during the first transfusion. Others followed. Within forty-eight hours, again displaying the extraordinary resiliency that had already sustained him beyond all expectation, John rallied.

Sunday afternoon, November 1, dressed in his pajamas and robe, he sat propped up in his hospital bed, on top of the blankets, absorbed in the morning comics. There was a light tap on the door. "May a little sister interrupt her brother's scholarly research?"

At the sound of the lyrical voice, John put down the paper. "Jill!" he said, delighted. "When did you get in?"

Wm. J. Buchanan

"Just an hour ago. Robert called last night and said you were ready to go partying."

During the first weeks following the discovery of John's illness, Robert and Jill experienced a despair they had never known. Both away from home, they longed for news of their brother, however small. They began to call home several times a week. Although John didn't complain, his parents noticed that the constant check-ups were unnerving him. Jack called Robert and Jill, explained the situation, and suggested they not call too often. From then on, he called them from his office to keep them abreast of John's condition.

By October 1970, his military commitment fulfilled, Robert and his family had returned to Albuquerque. He took over the job of keeping Jill informed.

Jill stepped over to the bed and gave her brother a hearty hug and kiss. "Let me look at you," she said. She stepped back a pace. With a wry chuckle she pointed to his feet. "Now where did you get *those!?*"

John's feet were covered by baby-blue, knit booties, decorated with matching toe-tassels. Sewn to the back of each bootie was a fluffy pom-pom pull-on tab. He wriggled his feet childishly. "One of my girls made them for me," he said with pride. "And I think they're elegant."

"That, they are." Jill laughed.

She looked up at the wall beside his bed. Attached there with surgical tape, a three-foot wide, ten-foot long single piece of heavy yellow paper, similar to that found on rolls in packaging departments of stores, stretched cater-cornered from the upper left ceiling to the opposite floor.

"What is that?" Jill asked. She stepped around the bed for a better look. Printed across the top of the long parchment were the words: "WE HOPE THIS MAKES YOU HAPPY." Directly beneath the heading and continuing down the entire length of the paper were hand-drawn or cut-out and pasted figures of children skipping rope, batting softballs, crouching to run, slapping at tether-balls, pumping swings, and engaging in other schoolyard activities. Scrawled at all angles over, under, beside and around the drawings were signatures of John's children.

Jill shook her head in wonder. "Why, there must be five hundred names there."

"Five hundred and seventeen," he replied proudly.

She stepped around the bed and pulled a chair close. They talked about the events in their lives since their last meeting. Good-naturedly, she fielded his questions about her welfare, recognizing that "big brother" was still protectively scrutinizing her life.

A half-hour later she rose to leave. "John, I must go. I've already overstayed my time."

John frowned. "Who says?" he asked, agitated.

"Your doctor says, that's who. It's for your benefit, and I'm going to listen to him."

"Oh, Jill!" he pleaded. "Come on. I'd much rather talk with you than read the funnies. Besides, I'm doing much better. Here, let me show you."

He swung his feet out over the side of the bed.

"John!" she cried in alarm.

He put a finger to his lips. "Sh-h-h-h!"

He put his feet on the floor, slowly shifted his weight to them and stood up. Clearly straining at the effort, he began a halting gait across the room, barely lifting his feet from the floor. At the door he grasped the jamb and held on tightly, breathing hard.

225

Thoroughly alarmed, Jill was tempted to rush to his side to help him. But something told her to let him continue this unexpected display unaided.

After a moment he let go of the door and started the same slow shuffle back across the room. At his bed he grabbed the headboard and leaned back against the frame, exhausted. He smiled feebly. "See!" he exclaimed. He was as excited as a child who had just won his first cross-country race.

Jill forced herself to smile. "John, that was wonderful!" Then she helped him into his bed, bent low, and kissed him on the cheek. "Now, John Baker, you rest. I'll be back every day."

He closed his eyes. She looked at him for a moment silently, then left the room and started down the hallway toward the elevator. Just past the nurses' station she spotted a waiting lounge. She entered the lounge and dropped into a chair. Her feigned smile had long since faded. No longer able to smother her emotions, she cried. Her brother had been so proud of proving to her that he could walk, barely, a mere twenty feet. *And this was a man*, she thought, *who once ran twenty-five miles a day!*

Gradually the combination of medication, transfusions and around-the-clock bedrest bolstered John's flagging strength to the barest level of self-mobility. Unable to roam the hospital corridors as he had before, he spent his time in his room. But the long hours were not wasted. For when he'd entered the hospital this time he had brought with him the ledger he had bought the day he had taken his mother to dinner at Coronado Center. Now, whenever he was without visitors, he spent his time writing in what was referred to by his family and friends as his "mysterious journal."

On November 10, thirteen days after the day he collapsed at Aspen, John was released from the hospital to go home.

Too weak now to risk himself behind the wheel of his cherished Triumph, but passionately determined not to meekly sit and wait for the end he knew was imminent, John enlisted his family and friends to keep him in touch with the meaningful interests of his ebbing life. Polly quit her job so she could tend to his needs. Day or night, she, Jack, Robert, John Haaland and a host of others stood ready to drive him any place he wanted to go.

Thursday afternoon, November 12, John sat on the couch in his living room gazing out the big picture window toward the Sandia Mountain. From a nearby chair, ostensibly reading, Polly watched him. His gaze was directed at the foothills that sheltered Aspen.

Every ten minutes he glanced at his watch, then back at the distant foothills. Shortly after three o'clock he looked over at his mother. "Mom, would you drive me somewhere?"

Polly got up from her chair. "Let me get a jacket."

John went to his room. When he came out, he was carrying his "mysterious journal."

"I'd like to go to Mrs. Mercer's office," he said. Polly now understood why her son had been glancing at his watch for the past hour. He wanted to go to Aspen before the Administration Offices closed, but after the children had left for home.

Veta Mercer greeted John warmly. Rising from her chair she stepped around her desk and took his hand. She was appalled at how much he had changed in the two weeks since she'd last seen him. His once flashing brown eyes were

227

dulled by sedatives. His color was pallid, a far cry from his once perpetual tan. And he moved slowly, pacing himself, she knew, to preserve what little strength he had left. But one thing had not changed—his winning smile.

"John!" Mrs. Mercer exclaimed. "What a pleasant surprise. Here, please sit down."

They talked for a while about his condition since the day she had helped him to the nurse's office following his collapse. Candidly, he told her he was now prepared for death at any moment. "To be truthful, Mrs. Mercer, that's why I'm here. Has the board selected my replacement yet?"

Mrs. Mercer paused. This was becoming a painful discussion for her. Yet, she sensed that for some reason he regarded it as business. She nodded. "Yes. Victor Moore."

John's eyes showed his pleasure. "Vic," he said reflectively. "Good. That's great."

Mrs. Mercer nodded. "I'm quite pleased with the choice."

He picked up the ledger he was holding in his lap and handed it across the desk. "Mrs. Mercer, would you please see that Vic gets this, and tell him it's from me."

Mrs. Mercer took the book from his hand.

"You may read it too," he said. "It's a coaching plan for my children. It'll give Vic a headstart with things it took me two years to learn. I thought that . . . well . . . it might make the transition easier. For him . . . and for them."

Mrs. Mercer opened the ledger and scanned through its many pages. It was a precise, detailed lesson plan geared to the children of Aspen. She noticed that the plan covered future semesters for '70–'71 and '71–'72—two complete school years.

She looked up at John. "I don't quite know what to say."

With considerable effort he pushed himself up out of his chair. "Just tell Vic to take care of my children, Mrs. Mercer."

Without another word he left the office. Veta Mercer never saw him alive again.

By mid-November, debilitated to the point where he could remain on his feet no longer than thirty minutes at a time, John at last realized that his hope of going to St. Louis was futile. During the week of November 15, with John Haaland or co-coach Pat Cox driving him, John attended every Duke City Dasher session, in the city or in the foothills, staying long enough each day to assure himself the lessons he had taught his girls were being put into practice.

Nights, he visited the Dashers a different way.

Each evening after dinner John went to the kitchen and pulled a chair close to the phone. For the next hour, or until exhaustion forced him to retire, he phoned the Dashers one by one. Following his coaching roster he kept up the calls until, over a peroid of a week, he had talked to all the girls who were scheduled to go to St. Louis, encouraging each to do her best in the finals.

On the night he called Jeanne Kroker he detected a note of distress in her voice.

"Jeanne," John said, "is something wrong?"

There was a pause. "Oh, Coach," the twelve-year-old girl said sadly, "I pulled a muscle in my leg at practice today. It hurts like crazy. I'm so afraid I won't get to go to the finals. And I want to so terribly much. But I know I can't take a seat on the plane if I won't be of any use to the team."

John knew the agony of missing a long-anticipated meet.

229

Wm. J. Buchanan

"Jeanne," he said at last, "there's going to be an empty seat on that plane. I want you to go to Saint Louis for me. If you can't run, give Coach Haaland as much help as you can, in my place."

"Hey, Coach!" Jeanne said. "Do you really mean that?"

"I mean it, honey. Just promise me one thing. Whatever you do—do your best."

"You bet I will!" the happy girl responded. "For you!"

Late Saturday night, November 21, Doctor Johnson put aside the book he was reading and glanced up at the clock on his den wall. It was nearing midnight. He was tired. But it was a good tired. He'd spent the day hiking in the foothills with his family, and now it was time for bed. He reached above his chair to turn off the reading light, just as the phone rang.

"Doctor," the answering-service operator said when he picked up the phone, "there's a Mrs. Baker on the line."

"Put her through," Johnson said.

Polly's voice was tense but controlled. "Doctor, John is doubled over in pain. It's the worst yet. But he begs us not to take him to the hospital."

"Is he fully conscious?" Johnson asked hastily.

"Yes."

"Take him straight to my office. I'll be there in fifteen minutes."

The Bakers' brown Oldsmobile had just pulled to a stop in the parking lot in front of Johnson's office when he drove up. As he turned off the engine, he could hear John's pathetic cries in the still night. Quickly, Johnson jumped out and ran to the Bakers' car. Behind the wheel, Jack was sitting with his body turned sideways, staring into the back

230

seat. There, like a babe-in-arms, John sat curled in his mother's lap. "Help me!" he sobbed. "Oh, my God-d-d-d! Won't somebody please help me-e-e!"

Her countenance a mask, Polly stroked her son's contorted face as she moved her body to and fro, slowly, in a maternal rocking motion.

"Loosen his trousers and pull them down!" Johnson ordered.

He wheeled and ran to his office. He unlocked the door, left it wide open and rushed to his drug-storage safe. Flicking on the light he opened the safe, grabbed a vial of Demerol and a hypodermic syringe. He filled the hypo, tested it, ran back to the Bakers' car and injected the needle into John's bare hip. In seconds the pain-relieving narcotic began to take effect. John's tormented body went limp in his mother's lap.

Without moving him, Johnson checked John's vital signs. After a moment Johnson looked at Polly and shook his head, "A few days at most," he said softly.

"He wants to stay at home," she replied evenly.

Johnson nodded. He closed the door and walked around to the driver's side of the car. "Mr. Baker," he said, "would you please wait a moment? I'll be right back."

He went into his office. In a few minutes he returned carrying a small snap-shut case. He opened the car door and handed the case to Jack. "This is a hypo of Demerol. It's all we can do now. Just inject it the way I showed you, whenever necessary. Don't hesitate to use it. and let me know so I can refill it."

For several seconds Jack stared at the hypo case. Finally he took it from Johnson's hand. "I understand," he said. He drove away without another word.

At 8:00 o'clock Sunday morning John awoke from a heavily drugged sleep and managed to get out of bed. He called his mother to his room. "Mom, please help me dress. I've got to go somewhere with Mr. Newton."

Without a murmur of protest Polly helped her son into his clothes. Twenty minutes later, after feeding him a meager liquid breakfast, she walked by his side, guarding him from falling, as he walked across the yard and entered the car of Dasher parent, Joe Newton.

For the next three hours, incredibly, John stayed on his feet at the Albuquerque International Airport arranging a public display honoring the Duke City Dashers. Prominently located in a huge picture window in the main lobby, the display was a montage of photos of the Dashers in action, victory headlines, a collection of earned medallions and a list of Dasher triumphs.

When the work was finished, John retreated to a near-by bench and looked at the display, reflectively, for a long time. Finally, he turned to Joe Newton, sitting at his side. "My girls will see that when they leave for Saint Louis Thursday," he said wistfully. "I hope it makes them proud."

It was John Baker's final trophy for his beloved Duke City Dashers.

Chapter 21

Monday, November 23, on his last day at home, John awoke from a groggy sleep with a growing pain in his back. He recognized the symptom all too well. Forewarned by Doctor Johnson, he realized that his kidneys, now victims of the rampaging cancer, were struggling to survive. Pushing on his elbows he raised up in bed and tried to put his feet over onto the floor. Unable to sustain the effort he fell back, exhausted.

"Bob!" he cried aloud.

At the kitchen table with his parents, Robert jumped from his chair and ran to his brother's room. For the past three days Robert had remained at his parents' house, night and day, to help take care of his rapidly failing brother.

Robert pushed the bedroom door open. John looked up at him helplessly. "Bob. Hot water. Hurry!"

Robert understood at once. With a swift movement he

leaned down and lifted John's emaciated body from the bed and balanced him on his feet. Draping one of John's arms across his shoulder, Robert helped him to the bathroom, removed his pajamas and lifted him into the tub.

Robert adjusted the hot and cold faucets until the stream of water filling the tub burned his hand.

"Turn off the cold!" John ordered.

Wincing at the thought, Robert closed the cold spigot and watched the steaming hot water rise around John's body. Anticipating his brother's next demand Robert rushed to the kitchen, filled his mother's largest pots and pans with water and set them on the stove to heat. He had performed this unnerving ritual repeatedly in the past few days and had never fully reconciled himself to it. In a few minutes he knew that his brother would begin to cry out for hotter and hotter water. It was the only palliative aside from brain-numbing Demerol that assuaged his pain.

For the next two hours Robert heated and poured scalding water into the tub. As always before during these strange bathroom sessions John appeared genuinely relaxed, lolling in the tub, as his body took on the vermilion hue of a boiled lobster.

At eleven o'clock there was a rap on the bathroom door. Polly stuck her head in. "John, Mrs. Wills is here. What airline are the Dashers taking Thursday?"

"Frontier," John replied.

A few minutes later Polly returned. "She'd like to talk about the schedule. Will you be out soon?"

John shook his head. "Mom, we took care of all that yesterday. John Haaland has a schedule and there's one on my desk. If she needs more I'll be happy to talk to her. But she's going to have to come in here. I'm not getting out of this tub."

Shortly after noon Robert lifted his brother from the tub, dried him gently and helped him to his room. A few minutes later, fully dressed, and holding onto Robert's arm for support, John walked into the living room and reclined in a propped up position on the couch.

"Can you eat something, John?" Polly asked.

"Maybe some juice, Mom."

She fixed a tray of orange juice, freshly blended carrot juice, milk and hot tea. One by one he tasted each. Deciding he really wanted the carrot juice he drank it slowly and asked for a refill.

At one o'clock the doorbell sounded. Jack answered. From his pallet on the couch John called out to the familiar figure standing at the stoop. "Hey, Coach! come on in."

Hugh Hackett stepped across the vestibule, greeted the Bakers in his genial, soft-spoken manner, then walked across the room to his one-time star runner.

Pleased with the visit of his college track mentor, John smiled. Together he and Hackett had made track history and their friendship was deep.

"How do you feel, John?" Hackett asked.

John chuckled. "Well, I don't think I'm ready for the starting line-up, Coach."

For the next fifteen minutes they relived past glories, John reminiscing with spirit. But the effort was visibly taxing him.

Noting the strain creeping into John's voice, Hackett rose from his chair.

"Hey . . . sit down, Coach," John pleaded. "We haven't even blasted the Trojans yet."

Hackett laughed. "You did a pretty good job of that the first time. No, I've got to leave. Besides, you look a little feverish."

Gently, Hackett reached over, placed his hand on John's brow and held it there for several seconds. With a solicitous nod he dropped his hand to John's shoulder and gave it a pat. "Take care, John."

Polly walked with Hackett to the door. As he stepped out onto the porch, he hesitated, then turned back to Polly. His face was anguished. "I hope that wasn't too obvious," he said apologetically. "But I just had to touch John one last time."

Throughout the early afternoon John catnapped on the couch. At three o'clock, during a period of apparently deep sleep, he began to moan. Suddenly, he opened his eyes wide, gritted his teeth tightly, and gasped, "The hypo, quick!"

Polly turned toward the cupboard where the hypodermic case lay. Jack was already there. Quickly, he opened the case, withdrew the syringe and ran to John's side. On the couch Robert held John's writhing body to keep him from falling onto the floor.

Throughout John's long ordeal, no one had suffered more than Jack. Unable to speak his feelings, recently, he had been leaving for his office earlier each day, and staying later, desperately seeking escape in overwork. It hadn't helped. As John's agony grew, so did Jack's. And in time a pain would take root in his being that would not diminish with the passing years.

Now, as Jack stood for a long moment staring at his agonized son, he made no move to inject the needle.

Robert looked up at his father. "Dad! The shot!"

At the cry Jack looked at Robert. Jack's face revealed a deep inner turmoil. "Robert," he said plaintively, "what if we make him an addict?"

Robert was flabbergasted. "An addict!? Dad, look at

236

him!'' On the couch, in his brother's arms, John moaned in pain.

Grimfaced, Jack lowered the hypo, grasped John's waist and plunged the needle into his buttock. Slowly, John's writhing ceased.

Robert laid his brother back on his pallet. Unmoving, Jack still stood staring at his sedated son. All at once the painful, unmistakable meaning of that moment hit Robert. His father had not—could not—face the reality that his eldest son was dying. Shaken, Robert felt his anger turn to empathy for this anguished man standing before him; the man who had lovingly guided him and nurtured him as a child; who had never failed to respond when his children were in need.

Overcome by compassion Robert stood and put his arms around his father's shoulder. "Dad, don't worry. We'll fight the addiction after we lick the cancer.''

Without moving his eyes from John's reclining figure, Jack nodded.

For the next three hours John remained unmoving on the couch while his family stayed at his side. At six o'clock Polly got up and started for the kitchen. "I'll fix us some sandwiches,'' she said.

She had no more than gotten the words out when John sat bolt upright on the couch. "Oh, no,'' he cried out. "It's all black . . . like the school yard!''

Before anyone could reach him he stood up and took several steps toward the hallway. As Jack and Robert rushed toward him, he grasped his back and fell heavily against the wall. Without a sound he slid down the wall onto the hallway floor. He lay on his back, unmoving, obviously in a coma.

Polly ran to the kitchen phone and glanced at the emer-

237

gency number she had posted there days before. She dialed the number and ordered an ambulance to come at once to transfer a comatose patient to the hospital. Next, she called Doctor Johnson. At last, the emergency chores taken care of, she rushed to her fallen son's side. She put her hand to his brow, then turned to her husband. "You'd better call Jill."

Fifteen minutes later, in mounting fury, Jack once again went to the door and stared down the dark street. "Polly," he said, rushing back inside, "I'm going to put him in the car!"

Polly shook her head. "Please, Jack. Just another minute or two."

There was a loud knock. Jack ran across the room and threw open the door. Working hastily now the ambulance crew strapped John to a rolling stretcher, pushed him out of the house and loaded him into the waiting ambulance. Polly crawled in after the stretcher and took a small jump-seat next to her son. Jack and Robert ran to the car to follow.

Suddenly, as the ambulance pulled away with the sirens blaring, John opened his eyes. "Mom," he called softly.

Polly leaned over the stretcher. "Yes, John."

"Mom, I can't see," he said in a low whisper. "Am I in an ambulance?"

"Yes. It's all right. We'll be at the hospital soon."

There was a pause.

"Mom."

"Yes."

"Make sure all the lights are flashing. I want to leave the neighborhood in style."

Doctor Johnson studied the hurried test results thoroughly. He was sitting at a barren metal desk in the emergency room of Presbyterian Hospital. On the table beside him John lay fully conscious but unmoving.

Johnson set the test results aside and pushed back his chair. He stepped over to John's side. Barely moving his head, John looked into Johnson's eyes.

Johnson laid a hand on John's shoulder. "John," he said softly, "do you remember our talk in December, about facing the inevitable?"

John nodded.

"Your time has come, John."

Without changing expression John continued to look at Johnson. After a moment he nodded again. "I'm ready." He took a deep breath. "Doctor." His voice was almost a whisper.

"Yes, John."

"Thank you for giving me the extra months."

Without a word Johnson squeezed John's shoulder, nodded, and left.

He walked across the hall to the waiting lounge. Through the glass partition in the door he saw Jack and Polly sitting together on a couch. They were holding hands. In nearby chairs were Robert, and John Haaland. Johnson pushed open the door and walked into the room. His face mirrored his deep sorrow. He stopped in front of the couch. "Have you called Jill?" he asked.

"She's on her way," Polly replied. "But she won't be able to make it until about three in the morning."

Johnson nodded. "I think she'll get here in time." He paused. "I hope you can find some comfort in knowing that John has talked to me often about his faith. He isn't afraid of death."

Polly rose and took Johnson's hand. He looked at her in

239

admiration. Once again, he realized, she was trying to comfort him. He shook his head sadly. "I just wish there was something more I could have done."

He turned and left the room without another word.

Chapter 22

The bedside vigil was constant.

Heavily sedated, with drainage tubes inserted in both nostrils to ease the pressure of the fluids invading his lungs and abdomen, John lay semi-conscious in a restricted private room. Around the clock, his family and closest friends took turns by his side, while others remained close by. In the halls and lounges of Ward Three a steady stream of John's admirers, fellow-teachers, students and their parents came by, hoping for a chance to say a final word to this dying young man who had touched their lives.

For sixty-two hours, lapsing at times into brief coma, John tenaciously refused to give up.

Tuesday afternoon and all day Wednesday, two at a time, the adult visitors and some of the older children were allowed to enter his room. Often unable to speak he greeted them with a pale but buoyant smile and a feeble squeeze with his hand.

Wednesday evening Bill Wolffarth came to the hospital. At the sight of his highschool coach John visibly perked up. He motioned Wolffarth near the pillow. "I hear you quit smoking," John whispered.

Momentarily surprised, Wolffarth quickly recovered. "That's right, old buddy. You always wanted me to."

John smiled. "Good. I'm glad." He drifted off into sleep.

Wolffarth shook his head in wonder. *How typical,* he thought. Even on his deathbed John's concerns were still on the welfare of others.

At midnight Wednesday, as she had each hour since she came on duty, the ward nurse took John's vital signs. Without a word to Jack or Robert, or John Haaland, who were in the room, the nurse left hastily. She went down the hall to the lounge where Polly and Jill were taking a brief respite from their attendance at John's side. "Mrs. Baker," the nurse said, "I think you should go back to see your son."

Quickly, Polly and Jill returned to John's side.

Still, despite his rapidly failing body, John doggedly held on to life. At 2:00 A.M. he called out softly, "Dad."

Jack rose and leaned over the bed. "I'm here, John."

John moved his hand slowly toward the edge of the bed. Jack took it quickly. For several seconds, without a word, father and son looked into each other's eyes. Then, once again, John drifted off into sleep.

Still holding John's hand, Jack sat back down in his chair. Though they hadn't spoken a word Jack knew that his son had just told him goodbye.

Shortly before dawn John Haaland rose from his chair and walked to the head of the bed. For two days and nights,

242

since he had met the ambulance that rushed John to the hospital, Haaland had remained at his friend's side, leaving only to catch a few hours of sleep at home. But now, in the early hours of Thursday, November 26, Haaland realized, reluctantly, that it was time to end his vigil.

Grasping Baker's hand Haaland leaned low over the bed. "John," he said softly, "can you hear me?"

Baker's eyelids fluttered. He nodded, barely.

"I've got to go now," Haaland said. His voice was strained with emotion. "We're taking the Dashers to Saint Louis today—as you predicted."

With a faint smile Baker nodded again and moved his lips in words Haaland couldn't understand.

Haaland bent lower. "I'm sorry, John. I didn't hear you."

Baker's lips moved again. "Take care . . . " he whispered ". . . of my girls." He squeezed Haaland's hand with all the grip he had left.

Gently, Haaland returned Baker's grip. "I will." With tears welling in his eyes Haaland gave Baker's hand a final squeeze and laid it back on the bed. Somberly, he turned and left his dearest friend for the final time.

Shortly before 7:00 A.M., the faint opalescent light of a new dawn filtered through the northside window directly behind Polly's back and fell, gently across John's bed. Sitting at her son's left side Polly leaned her head forward onto the bed with her forehead resting lightly against his arm. Suddenly she was distracted from her reverie by a strange gurgling noise. Looking up, she saw one of the drainage tubes in John's nostrils turn from dark to brilliant red. She knew that meant the tumor had finally broken through to his lungs. With grim determination she lowered

243

her head again. "Dear God," she prayed aloud, "please grant my son peace."

Then she heard a faint whisper. "Hey . . . somebody's mother."

She looked at John who had turned his head on the pillow. He looked directly into her eyes. He held the gaze for several seconds. Then, whispering softly, he said, "I can't fight any longer. I'm sorry to have been so much trouble." With a final sigh John Baker closed his eyes forever.

It was Thanksgiving Day, 1970, eighteen months since he had first visited Doctor Johnson. He had defeated death by twelve months. He was twenty-six years old.

For several minutes Polly remained at the bedside gazing at her son's now peaceful face. It was over. At last she stood and turned to her grieving family. She looked from one to the other; her husband, her two remaining dear children. After a moment, her voice strong and even, she said, "This is truly Thanksgiving Day. John is no longer suffering."

Word of John's death spread quickly to the radio and television stations and thence throughout the city. It reached Albuquerque International Airport just as the Duke City Dashers were boarding their plane for the journey to St. Louis. Amid muffled cries the sad news was passed among the girls from seat to seat. All at once a car pulled alongside the loading plane. Robert Baker jumped from the car and ran up the loading ramp.

Gathering the Dashers at the rear of the plane. Robert confirmed the news they had already heard. "My brother won't be with you in person this trip," he told the heartbroken girls. "But he'll be with you in spirit. And he'll want you to do your best."

Minutes later as the lumbering prop-jet revved its engines and began taxiing toward the end of the runway for take-off, Jeanne Kroker reached down, unwrapped an ace bandage from her knee and began to flex her leg. Her seatmate regarded her with concern. "You don't have to do that, Jeanne. He'd understand why you can't run."

Through tearstained eyes Jeanne looked back at her seatmate. "Nothing," Jeanne said hoarsely, "can stop me from running now."

Two days later, with tears streaming down their cheeks, the Duke City Dashers won the National AAU championship in St. Louis—"for Coach Baker."

Chapter 23

The funeral was one of the largest in New Mexico history.

In a bronze casket draped with his cherry and silver UNM letter blanket, dressed in his green Duke City Dasher blazer, John's body lay amid a sea of flowers at the high altar of Central United Methodist Church, where only a short time before he and James Hawk had so often prayed together in the final weeks of their lives. In the audience 1500 people lined the pews, the aisle, and stood crowded around the walls. Over half of them were "John's children."

Left of the aisle, across from the Baker family, the victorious Duke City Dashers, resplendent in their green uniforms, filled the front rows. Behind them, with their parents, were the children of Aspen, many of them touched by death for the first time. Near-by were Stephanie Keel, and

247

John's "student assistant coaches"—Bill Witherspoon, Anthony Straquadine, Chuck Lander, Ron Jones and Bobby Abeyta.

The audience stood and bowed their heads as the Reverend Doctor Harry Vanderpool intoned John's favorite Biblical passage, from St. Paul's second letter to Timothy:

> The time of my departure has come,
> I have fought the good fight. I
> have finished the race.

During the file past the bier, which took two hours, Doctor Johnson laid his hands on top of John's, and wept openly.

That afternoon, Monday, November 30, borne by his coaches and former teammates, and flanked by the Dashers and the children of Aspen, John's body was laid to rest in Sandia Memorial Gardens, high on the East Mesa, in the shadow of towering Sandia Peak. At his head a flush-mounted granite stone was set in place bearing the simple inscription by which he wished to be remembered:

COACH
JOHN W. BAKER
1944–1970

But the John Baker story does not end in death.

The day following John's funeral a phenomenon began at Aspen. En masse, the children began to refer to the school as "John Baker School." Within days no student would refer to the school by its real name. "It's our school," they told their astonished parents and teachers, "and we want to call it 'John Baker.'"

Impressed by their children's fervor, a parents' group was formed to officially suggest the name change to the Albuquerque Board of Education.

The board was skeptical. Uncertain about how the change would be accepted by the district as a whole, the board recommended a referendum and promised to abide by a majority vote.

The following April, 520 families in the Aspen School District voted on the question. There were 520 votes for; none against.

On May 16, 1971, in an impressive ceremony attended by the top school officials of the city, hundreds of John's friends, his family and all of "his" children, his UNM letter blanket, encased in glass, was mounted on the wall of the multipurpose room at Aspen where he had once taught. His track shoes, bronzed for preservation, and the remainder of his medals and trophies, were encased near-by. Then, by unanimous proclamation of the Albuquerque Board of Education, Aspen School officially became John Baker Elementary. It stands today as a fitting monument to a courageous young man who, in his darkest hours, transformed bitter tragedy into an enduring legacy.